MW01401531

I Ordered *My* Future Yesterday

I Ordered *My* Future Yesterday

The Julie Cox Story

JULIE COX

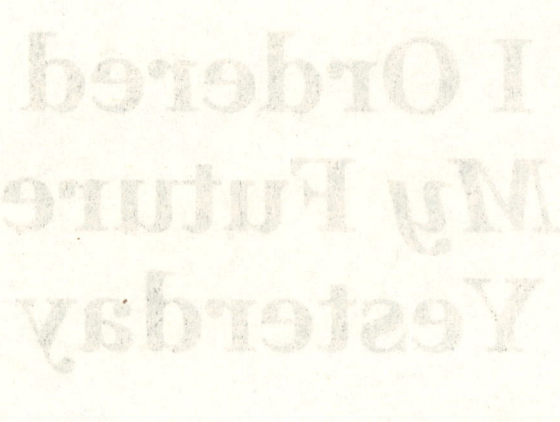

Order this book online at **www.trafford.com**
or email orders@trafford.com

Most Trafford titles are also available at major online book retailers.

Printed in the United States of America.

ISBN: 978-1-4269-7458-8 (sc)
ISBN: 978-1-4269-7459-5 (hc)
ISBN: 978-1-4269-7460-1 (e)

Library of Congress Control Number: 2011911167

Trafford rev. 08/30/2011

www.trafford.com

North America & International
toll-free: 1 888 232 4444 (USA & Canada)
phone: 250 383 6864 • fax: 812 355 4082

CONTENTS

“This sad story details a young woman's journey from her childhood in a very poor home in the Philippines to an adulthood that brings her back to the Philippines but now as a wealthy, yet charitable business owner. She experienced many obstacles along the way, including multiple rapes, years of scrounging through a garbage dump for food, leukemia, other severe illnesses, and perhaps the most heart-breaking decision to give up her six-year-old for adoption. All through these traumas, she kept her faith and her desire to make her life worthwhile—and she has. As an autobiography, it gives personal details that only she could bring to life including her struggles, rewards, and finally the discovery of her earthly soul mate. This story uses bible verses and tragic events to inspire true hope.

The author puts her most personal details in print in an effort to tell the reader that no matter how bad they think they have it, it could be worse. She doesn't sugar coat her struggles, but employs them for positive lessons. Her writing style is kept simple with examples of pop culture, including songs and TV characters—most likely in an attempt to lighten the very heavy subject matter. The author is reflective of her Catholic beliefs on almost every page and never misses an opportunity to inject spiritual insight. It's a good story, with gratefully a happy ending, although it might employ more precise details of her childhood to adult transition. It is a story of miracles, faith, and love that leaves the reader both thankful and reflective.”

Jenifer Kimble
The US Review of Books

"Though terrible tragedies happen, survival is for those who continue to live despite the darkest of days. This is the recurring theme in *Julie Cox's I Ordered My Future Yesterday: The Julie Cox Story*. Cox herself has suffered through many dark times, from intense poverty in the Philippines to rape, pregnancy from the rape, and leukemia- all by the age of twenty-four. However, her book is not a collection of depressing tales. Instead, it celebrates the author's ability to fight her way past, her circumstances and find success, happiness and redemption. Not only does Cox survive her traumatic experiences, but she finds ways to make life better for others along the way. She searches for and finds the child she put up for adoption. She provides assistance to disadvantaged kids for their education. She regains the land her father gambled away. Cox prefers to teach and inspire rather than live in the past. She begins her book with "Fifteen Keys to Life." Here, she shares the wisdom she has gained from her life experiences. For example, she writes that, "The light of a brighter future can be seen through even the smallest hole." Her positive outlook in the face of much adversity is what makes the book so special and inspirational. At no point in her writing does Cox sound angry or depressed. Instead of playing the blame game or cursing the world, she invites readers to "Dare to Dream."

The chapters of *I Ordered My Future Yesterday* are so packed, Though, that sometimes lose focus. If key events and images were presented in a more organized fashion, the book would be more effective. Still, the author's message shines."

Foreword Clarion Review
A Four Stars Review

"Proof: The giver is the gift." This is a very difficult book to Review. Not that it is good or bad but more than that it is stirring, heart-wrenching and compelling in ways that are difficult to describe and that would do the book the "justice" it is worthy of.

I wanted to put the book down after reading the chapter "The Gospel According to Leukemia" but was not able to. I had to know more about the courage and undaunted spirit of the Author, Julie Cox.

I don't think I've ever read a book that provided more reasons where "giving up" seemed like the thing to do and Julie on several occasions wanted to do just that but was saved in miraculous ways that surprised even her! I was mortified only to later be cheering, Julie, on back again, to anguish and heartache, to unbelievable joy, as this incredible woman doesn't just "overcome" trials but breaks through them with power, determination and a humble, grace that is so transformative I was completely caught up in, not the story but the "life" of this remarkable woman. Over and over again, Julie defies all odds and only comes back more determined and always with a generous heart.

Julie's story is not a story of overcoming as it is a story of discovery of her own unique nature which in every case desires to return to others what was given to her. Here is a woman who, in her life experience and in her own words, "has overcome the world".

In every way, this book is a gift as is Julie. Her story truly is evidence that the greatest gifts in life are those that are returned from the abundance we all have within. Julie's faith, courage, perseverance and love of family and life is the greatest testament that regardless of what life throws at us, an indomitable spirit and generous heart always triumphs. I want to carry her on my shoulders and parade here around for all to see just as all "heroes" should be.

Carl Bozeman
Author
AMAZON BESTSELLER
"On Being God- Beyond Your Life's Purpose
Are you Listening? Addressing the Divine Within
On Human Being- Loving and Living without Purpose"

Here's an unparalleled story of a Filipina Cinderella whose glass slippers for once shoeless Julie represent marginalization and hard toil that turned one's unrelenting passion to compassion. What I salute in the author's story is the multiplicity of misfortunes that fortified the walls of her heart and kept her soul pure and unblemished, open to look out not only for the salvation of her immediate family and clan but now the rest of the world. In my personal encounter with Julie, I have no doubt that she is a true missionary both in word and in deed.

Marita De Guzman Viloria, PhD
Founder KALINGA CROSSOVER MISSION

Acknowledgement

I wish to thank Anthony LoBaido for editing the first phase of this book.

I am very fortunate to have met and worked with David Flannery, Trafford Senior Publishing Consultant.

His encouragement and firm belief in this book inspired me to have the soaring spirit to share my complete life story and the longings of my heart and soul.

I am also grateful to the entire Trafford Publishing team for making my dream come true, to have a book that can inspire readers and give praise to the Lord.

Dedication

This book is for the glory of God for resurrecting my life and for all the blessings He bestowed upon me and my family.

He is the Light I follow.

My husband Lou, for standing by me through the years, giving me hope and a shoulder to cry on during difficult times.

For my son, Armand Joey, the recipient of my endearing unconditional love.

Julie Cox is no ordinary woman. Born in the Philippines, she's carved out an amazingly fruitful life after overcoming a plethora of obstacles that would have broken a lesser person. In her new book, *I Ordered My Future Yesterday*, Julie recounts the trials and tribulations she's faced, including being raped twice and left for dead, extreme poverty, the death of various loved ones, and giving up the baby she had after being raped the second time for adoption.

Julie will take you with her as she recounts how she lived for two years scavenging as a semi-orphan amid a garbage dump at the US Naval Base at Subic Bay. Follow her as she tells how she moved from the Philippines to the United States and began a series of odd jobs that in turn led to a successful sales career. During this time, Julie remained busy building her dream resort and academic training center in the Philippine Islands piece by piece. And now, through sheer hard work and crafty planning, she's halfway toward being a millionaire.

You'll learn about how she was stricken with leukemia as a teenager, how she contracted infectious hepatitis, and how she was put in nearly solitary confinement (alone and without visitors) at a government hospital in Manila for months on end. She also endured abuse and cruelty every step of the way. She went through issues with her son and his illness and a painful separation from him for fourteen years. You will learn what happened when they finally encountered each other again.

As an immigrant to the United States, Julie is more American than the blonde next door—more than any —sweet young thing from Indiana." This is because she embodies the character traits many average Americans lost long ago—love, honor, backbreaking labor, honesty, sacrifice, and courage. Through her faith, Julie expresses her desire to overcome the world, the flesh, and the pride of life while seeking to bring glory to God by using her talents in His service and in the service of others.

Most important, Julie details her philosophies and inspirations, drawing a comprehensive picture of what it takes for people to overcome the many obstacles they may face in life—be they mental, spiritual, physical, or emotional.

This is the journey and the adventure from the darkest corners of the human psyche to the narrow road that leads to peace, joy, contentment, and fulfillment in our troubled world. There are plenty of feel-good books out there. Yet in this short but poignant true-life fairy tale, Julie shows readers they must never give up. Most importantly, Julie Cox demonstrates it's not about feeling good or looking good; it's about being good.

From *I Ordered My Future Yesterday*

"On the other side of my midnight is morning. Yet sometimes it's the other way around. Sometimes on the other side is a place awaiting darkness, and I have to find my 'light' all over again."

"I was so broken many times. It was so unreal that this could happen to the same person so many times. During my teenage years, I didn't have any boyfriends—zero! But it was like I had a huge sign in my body saying, 'Abuse me.' I was raped at fifteen and then again when I was twenty-four years old. I had my son as a result of that, and he became sickly like I was."

"If certain men thought I was "hot" well, I can tell you that they made me feel totally 'cold' through their wicked behavior and actions via the multiple rapes."

"Only my younger sister knew where my son and I were. We were up in the mountains hiding with scavengers at the former Subic Naval Base. We couldn't come home, as my mother had disowned me in shame. My younger sister supported us all she could with her salary, but we just could not survive the illness and hunger, so we had to come home to my other sister in Manila."

"There was more hardship than you can imagine. The living conditions were not good. My son developed chronic bronchitis and was always having lung infections. I myself was so sickly that I wished not to live anymore. I couldn't focus on God. I thought He was punishing me for all these things I did not deserve, including having a son out of wedlock. I believed this even though I had been raped and was not morally at fault."

"I loved my son so much that I asked God to take my life if it would save my son from agony because of his illness. He was not breathing when his asthma attacked. I died (metaphorically) every time it happened. My eyes were never dry. My eyes were a true bucket of tears."

"This was my life, day after day ..."

I alone know the plans I have for you. Plans to bring you prosperity and not disaster. Plans to bring about the future that you hope for.

—Jeremiah 29:11

About the Writing of This Book

When Julie Cox approached me about writing and editing her life story, I knew immediately that I would try to "stay out of the way" and let her tell the tale. What you are about to read is her story—purely, totally, and fully. I merely edited the lexis and copy. I tried to make it flow. I fixed mistakes, added a few words here and there, and organized the chapters. I tried to clarify what was unclear through further interaction with Julie.

Although Julie and I have been acquainted for three years, I only knew bits and pieces of her tale. Now for the first time, I am putting together the full story of my friend. I believe she has shown courage, honor, and kindness.
In life, when you are knocked down as Julie has been, you have to find the courage to stand back up like in the *Rocky* movies. Julie shows the reader a rare glimpse at what it means to have almost limitless courage.

Of course, a project of this magnitude is not without many obstacles. To begin, English is not Julie's first language. Her first language is Tagalog, which is what they speak in the Philippines. She only went to school up to the seventh grade. During the time I was asked to edit this book, I slipped in the pouring rain and fell down two flights of stairs, separated my shoulder, and wound up in a sling.

Thus every keystroke and every action involved intense pain. This in some ways brought me closer to Julie and the pain she had endured.

Since I edited the book on Ko Pha Ngan Island off the coast of southern Thailand, we were subject to an impromptu and unscheduled monsoon season (during what should have been the dry season), frequent power outages, and no running water for up to a week at a time. Of course, I was propelled forward by the positive feedback I received about the book from many friends around the world, especially Robert Charette, a full-blooded Lakota American Indian and ex-special forces operator with the US Army, and my mentor, Dr. Loyal Gould, a giant of the journalism establishment. Dr. Gould craftily told me to "strike while the iron is hot."

As for Julie, she is obviously not a journalist and had to face the prospect of recalling all she had been through in life—the rapes, the trauma, the abandonment, the separation, health issues, and many other things—virtually all at once. This was overwhelming at times for her. She showed (again) moxie, bravery, and a willingness to face her darkness.

I must admit, reading and editing what Julie wrote also drove me closer to the Lord and inspired me. This is why I continued to edit and rewrite the book even with a dislocated shoulder and little or no sleep. Thus it is my deepest honor to tell her story. The writing of this book was one of Julie's dreams. Now that dream has become a reality. Praise God!

– Anthony C. LoBaido

Preface:
The Fifteen Keys to Life

1) Believe in God. Everything happens for a reason. What sometimes breaks us makes us stronger, and in the end your strength will be unbreakable under any circumstances.

2) You can rise above your trials and tribulations. You will find your strength. The light of a brighter future can be seen through even the smallest hole.

3) Believe in yourself so others may also believe in you, and so they might begin to believe in themselves.

4) Dare to dream! Your dreams are your shining stars. If you believe, your star will guide you which way to go. Dreams are your future discovered, so always act on your dreams.

5) Love your parents, and be grateful under any circumstances for all they have done for you. They gave you life, and you are here for a reason—maybe even a divine reason.

6) Have a sense of responsibility for yourself and society. Be not a burden but a proud, patriotic citizen of your country.

7) Be an instrument of change for the benefit of yourself and others. If you help yourself and become successful, then you can help others with your generosity.

8) Promote peace, love, and charity. God will measure your good works one day.

9) Promote the love of nature and the environment. Your children and the children of your children will remember and benefit from your sensibilities.

10) Prosperity is not only material wealth. Generosity of kindness and compassion to others also enrich our souls.

11) Give until it hurts. You will be rewarded to the same measure as you give.

12) Make sacrifices for the good of others and not for self-interest and/or glorification.

13) Be a bridge over troubled waters. Lend a hand to someone having difficult times.

14) The sun always shines the brightest after heavy storm. Whatever you think is your worst problem, somebody else has it worse than you do. You will always see the light is brighter after going through the darkness.

15) Metaphorically, heaven can be a parallel realm on earth just as well. You can find it when you find the ways needed to make other people happy. Heaven can thus be found in people‘s smiles of gratitude aimed back at your simple kindness shown toward them.

What If ...

I've often wondered, "What if ...?"

What if my father hadn't gambled away all his real estate inheritance?

My parents probably would have been able to send me to school beyond the seventh grade, and I would most likely have finished my education.

I would have stayed in the Philippines, not come to America, and would have met a man, married, and had children.

My life would just probably be just ordinary—no sufferings, no sacrifices, and perhaps not worth living in the extraordinary sense.

Yet my life has been extraordinary, a miracle that has been fully examined.

My soul is full of scars, yet I know in my heart I will face my Maker with a smile on *His* face. I will not faint. I will run the race. I will see the Lord's approval and His face always.

I wouldn't have learned to devote my life toward spiritual things like giving time and money to the poor. Because of my past sufferings, I learned how to be compassionate to the needy. It gives me so much joy to share and give until it hurts. I sold my "precious" jewelry in time for my recent birthday in order to buy groceries for the indigent people in my barrio back in the Philippine Islands (PI). Those people are truly precious.

I wouldn't probably have been able to appreciate the value of learning God's wisdom.

Wisdom from God has made the years of my life fruitful and profitable.

I probably wouldn't know that forgiveness is a gift to myself, not only set aside for those people who have hurt
me.

As Anthony C. LoBaido says (and I realize I should be chastised on many fronts for quoting him so often, but he has such amazingly intense and wonderful wisdom), "We cannot judge or punish ourselves or others . Only God is fit to do that."

When I chose to forgive, that is when God starts my healing. Then all of my hurts became my "jewels" I can take to heaven. We must store our treasure in heaven, for this world and everything in it is passing away, just as the Bible teaches us.

So I ask "What if ...?" but not without having the Lord show me, "Why and what for?"

Plato's advice remains true: "An unexamined life is not worth living." God, not man or his high technology, is the measure of all things.

Why This Book, Julie?

The writing of this book has long been one of my dreams. I was told that I must not be afraid of this book. Of course I had my doubts. As you've already heard, my native language is Tagalog, which sounds a bit like Spanish and is the preferred language of the PI. English is my second language. I only went to school until the seventh grade. That's two major strikes against me.

But I believe, for some reason I cannot fully comprehend, that it's God's will for me to write my life story with His help. I waited and waited upon the Lord, and then I finally asked Anthony C. LoBaido to write it for and with me. Could I face the pain of my rapes, sicknesses and so many other things all over again? Would doing this be of value to others? Would it bring God glory? In the macro sense, my dreams include helping others, building a school, and devoting my life to the service of the Lord.

We should never give up before our miracles happen. We should seek to overcome our near misses. We should all "order our futures" and expect them to arrive right at our doorstep at the proper moment. "Always best, and by doing so you will let loose some kind of special and mystical power from yourself ..." This is indeed the power of positive thinking in the finest sense. But positive thinking without real action is empty.

On the other side of my midnight is morning, yet sometimes it's the other way around. Sometimes waiting on the other side is a place and I have to find my "light" all over again.

Yes, *la vida es una puta entonces*. We find pieces that fit after the storm. Life is difficult sometimes. Are we unknowingly punishing ourselves for our sins? Is it a test like that experienced by Job? Are we in judgment like Jonah inside the whale?

Recollecting the "unwanted debris" of my past causes me (at times) to go into a downward spiral of emotion. Of course, at times I've had second thoughts about why I'm punishing myself by recounting this. For what reason am I doing this? It's certainly not for the money, because there are so many spiritual, motivational, feel-good books out there already.

No, rather it's because there's an inner voice telling me I should make this book a reality. Indeed, the inner voice is telling me I should do this book (Anthony has told me this again and again and again) because there is someone "out there"—a lost and broken soul—who will be "found" and perhaps even inspired by reading my story.

As Emily Dickenson said, "If I can stop one heart from breaking, I shall not live in vain."

In a similar style, I will say only this: If I can save one soul from wandering off from God's grace, perhaps there will be rejoicing and happiness in heaven. It is my great hope that this book will do just that.

With God's help I've relived all of this pain for you, dear reader. How did I do this?

Philippians 4:13 tells us, "I can do all things through Christ who strengthens me."

I know it's just one verse from the Bible. I realize my life can't be summarized in one quotation, nor can it be abbreviated, as it is all from the wisdom of God.

Yet I believe that my life is best explained by reading Jeremiah 29:11: "I alone know the plans I have for you. Plans to bring you prosperity and not disaster, plans to bring about the future that you hope for."

All of my life's trials and tribulations are part of God's perfection in my life. I am grateful for the opportunity to have shared in His cross. I've known suffering because He wanted me to have strength and perseverance. By not giving up, we can find God's approval. The Bible says, "Whoever does not take up the cross and follow Me is not worthy of Me."

I've known trials and challenges in life. And why not? Jesus Christ was also prosecuted for crimes He did not commit. How blessed I am to have the opportunity to feel and know what real love and real victory are. No servant is greater than his or her master. The poet Robert Browning wrote, "For sudden the worst turns the best to the brave." We must have faith and walk in the power of Jesus Christ.

When I say love, it is love coming from God, for God is love. Everything that is most meaningful in my life comes through the goodness of the Lord. Everything that is coursing through my veins is of God. My strength is God. Because of my belief and faith in Him, He does not fail me. Everything is made possible in my life because of God.

If you believe in Him and do not waver, He will give you what you are praying for. If you focus on God, then He will focus on you. Work and pray continually, try to be good, and do good things for others. Then one day He will show you the way to God's kind of prosperity and most importantly, the way to heaven.

God has a plan for me. It is a plan that can be seen only by Him. I would have not seen this plan if He hadn't broken me. My brokenness has reasons that go far beyond what I can ever imagine. Now I can detail what's long been written in my heart of hearts.

As the often-embattled, late former President Richard M. Nixon said, "Only if you have been in the deepest valley can you imagine how magnificent it is to be in the highest mountain."

I once lived in a garbage dump. I was struck down with leukemia. I was raped. I was raped again and left for dead. As a result of that rape, I became pregnant. Most people would have had an abortion within society's moral reasoning. I did not. I took that violence and evil and turned it into life with God's help. I can say my spirit soars because God turned all of these sufferings and trials and evils into an unimaginable life of goodness and triumph.

Chapter 1

In the Beginning

Life was just so hard when I was growing up in the Philippines.

My earliest years were not happy ones. My youth was misspent on many worries and problems centered on extreme poverty. I cannot recall any happy moments from my childhood and teen years. I know that's kind of sad to say, but that's the way it was.

I was the ninth child of twelve. My father was a village carpenter. My mother was just a traditional Filipina subservient wife doing everything humanly possible to take care of all of us. We were like a small army. As Napoleon noted, an army travels on its stomach. Napoleon also said, "Let China sleep, for when she awakes, let the nations tremble." What he didn't say was, "A walk is as good as a hit."

I would tell Napoleon that while I'm not quite sure exactly what he meant by his most-famous quotes, I've trembled and I've been hit time and time again. My stomach has often ached for even the smallest morsel of food. Have you ever been truly hungry even one day of your life?

Back to my loving mother ... all of the housework was done manually—laundry, cooking by firewood, and so forth. And let me tell you that fetching water from the well took forever and a day. A woman's work is never done. These never-ending tasks made my mother a spent woman, tired and haggard all of the time. It was very sad to witness. It left an indelible impression upon me, so much so that I vowed I would never get married.

I recall many sad moments when I was only about seven years old. My father would go to buy lumber and other materials for his house-building contracts and would not come home for days on end. It would happen many times. I saw the heartbreaking spectacle of watching my mother cry because she would have to send me to the neighbors to borrow rice, as we didn't have any food in the pantry. If a burglar had broken into our house, we would have robbed the burglar. That's how poor we were!

Later on I learned that my father would gamble all the money away to no end, even until there was no more money for his bus fare. When he did come home, he would work until the wee hours to pay off his gambling debts and had very little left for our food and bare necessities. It was like *Of Mice and Men*, only instead of George and Lenny, one smart guy and one stupid guy, we had two stupid guys—my father and the mystery man who took over his body to start gambling. I swear if we lived in Las Vegas, my father would have become the second coming of Wayne Newton and never left the place.

Meanwhile, all my older brothers and sisters capable of working in different factories in Manila left to help support my mother and us younger brothers and sisters.

The sad part was although my older brothers and sisters were very smart academically, none of them went past the sixth grade in school. As I noted, they all had to go to different places to find work. You might think all of this is like something out of a Charles Dickens novel, but this was our reality. We were not the *Partridge Family*. This was not *Family Guy* or the *Simpsons*. This was hardcore poverty. This was the result, in part, of sin.

Wasn't Jesus Christ Himself and His father Joseph a carpenter? Didn't Joseph, Jesus's earthly father, take Mary and Jesus into the deserts of Egypt to avoid the assassins sent by a local jealous king? This had to have been the ultimate special forces mission ever attempted in human history. The whole fate of humanity rested on the shoulders of one carpenter moving by stealth from Bethlehem to Egypt. God trusted a carpenter with this.

Was our father gambling with our very lives? This is the result of a life of sin and temptation—to gamble for what ... a cheap thrill? Where is the satisfaction in that compared with building a house or a barn or a den or a library, something that will last years or generations that you can take real pride in? Why didn't my father look at life in this way? He wasn't using "the Force" like in Star Wars. He wasn't in the special forces. He was a disaster waiting to happen. I never really understood why.

But make no mistake about this fact—my father was a very kind and generous man. He was even considered a genius and partly a medicine man, as he often cured himself of various illnesses. He is a Roman Catholic, and although he seldom goes to church, his philosophies and words of wisdom come from the Bible.

Sadly, his pitfall was his gambling compulsion, and he lost all of his inherited real estate properties. It can be looked upon as a sad tale that we learned about through my mother's constant conversation with us on the matter. She always said we could have all gone to school if my father hadn't gambled away our collective and individual futures.

I'd always dreamed of going to school and learning beyond my years. I was always in the top of my class from first to the fourth grade. I went to school with no books and sometimes no pencil or paper—and most of the time with no slippers or shoes. I was "the little girl with no shoes." I will never forget when I heard there was a famous baseball player over a century ago called "Shoeless Joe Jackson." I was "Shoeless Julie."

But Shoeless Joe took off his baseball cleats in the outfield (according to baseball folklore) because they were uncomfortable for his feet. They said "his glove was where triples went to die." I like that phrase because that is how God, His angels, and the Holy Spirit operate, like fleet centerfielder Rick Ankiel running down all of the spiritual hits that might smash us.

Sometimes we crash into a wall chasing down fly balls or even false dreams. I had a dream of a normal life. I suppose those American soldiers marching through the Bataan Death March also had future dreams. I don't mean to complain. Look at the people in Cambodia stepping on land mines. A handful do so each and every day.

Food was always more important to my family than education, and as far as my father was concerned, as long as I knew how to read and write, that was sufficient. He figured girls just end up getting married anyway. Again, as noted, I made a vow to myself, believe it or not, that I would never get married, and at that time I was only eight years old.

My mother would always scrounge and provide money for my school necessities, but I knew it was very, very difficult for her. This situation left an indelible mark on my consciousness and later the pact I made with myself, namely that I would never forget little children, like myself, with no shoes and to help schoolchildren who can‘t afford school supplies.

These days I buy them in bulk and send them back to the needy in the Philippine Islands as frequently as I can. I don‘t want a medal. I don‘t want praise. I just want to bring God glory by serving others. We are not saved by works, but we must show good fruit. This so God will tell us in the end, “Well done, my good, and faithful servant.”

Anyway, at night back in those days I prayed to God and wished upon a shooting star that some stroke of good luck would happen that we would somehow get out of poverty. To be perfectly honest, sometimes I thought that maybe God had forgotten us, like Joseph of old in Egypt must have felt, stripped of his coat of many colors. So I would pray, look at the shooting stars up in the sky, and ask, “God, why is this happening? Why are things like this? Where are you, God?”

I know being poor is not a sin, and I was not ashamed of our deplorable situation. However, I thought that if God truly loved my family, perhaps we would not be so very poor. I also think perhaps we were rich in other ways. Former Vice President Dan Quayle sometimes spoke of a “poverty of values." I heard he also couldn't spell the word potato correctly. Oh how I longed for a potato at times back in those days.

During my fifth grade year, I had to go to another school, as the village school I attended only went up to fourth grade. The elementary school was five kilometers each way from home. (A kilometer is .6 miles.) I would get up at dawn, cook my food, and then walk barefoot to school every day, rain or shine. I would cross the flooded river when it was heavy monsoon season, arrive home wet, muddy, and exhausted, and then do it all over again. This went on for the next two years until I graduated from the sixth grade.

Despite all the hardships and the fact that there was plenty I couldn't count on in life, I made it through graduation with honors. It was one of the happiest moments of my life when my mother walked up to the stage with me and pinned a ribbon of honor upon me. At that particular moment, I knew what I wanted to be. I wanted to write, and I wanted to take lovely pictures of many beautiful places in the world.

Back then I had yet to look up in the dictionary just exactly what a photojournalist was. But all along that is what I wanted to become. Little did I know I would have the opportunity later on in life to learn photography and carry out my own writing projects.

— — —

At a very young age, I was different. I was mature for my age, and I had lofty ambitions. Despite my poverty, I believed I could still rise up. I believed I could fly and that I could reach for the sky. Dreams do have the capability to create miracles in your life.

But a major disappointment broke my heart to pieces after my sixth-grade graduation. I was told by my mother and father I would not be able to continue my education to high school, as they could not afford the matriculation fees, books, uniform, and shoes. (As if I needed shoes. I mean, come on! I was Shoeless Julie, roaming the outfield of life.)

It was devastating for me, and I cried for weeks. My heart became so sick and very sad. I became sickly and depressed. I became mad that God made us poor, and I even thought in those weak moments that God had forsaken me as His child. I went through loneliness and depression seeing my classmates go by to school every day.

Now and then when I remember those days, I have to find ways to help some students who are in need. Again, I can't stress this enough, those very sad experiences made me compassionate to the needy. How can I ever forget?

I now have a medical and dental mission every year at my resort. Of course it is free for indigent people. Always I hold this event on my birthday as a gift of appreciation to *God* for resurrecting my life.

My older brother as well as my sister, who both could have helped me go to school, eloped and married simultaneously, so I lost all my hope of going to school. I was back in the gutter. The star I was looking to become was far away indeed. I was the sun, and my stardom was Proxima Centauri, the next closest star to our sun. I don't know how far away it is, but it's really far—light years kind of far.

Another year passed, and my brother decided to bring me to Manila and got me a job at a hosiery mill. At the same time, I was also his babysitter-housekeeper. I was overworked and overtired all the time. I was extremely anemic and would pass out constantly. When my brother finally took me to the hospital and did all the blood work, my diagnosis was summed up in one word.

That word wasn't, "Oh, she needs some vitamins." No, not for Julie; it was "fatal." The doctors told me that I had something called leukemia. They told me I was going to die.

But you know something? God wasn't going to let me die, because God had big plans for me, just as He has big plans for you, my dear reader.

Remember again Jeremiah 29:11: "I alone know the plans I have for you. Plans to bring you prosperity and not disaster, plans to bring about the future that you hope for."

Chapter 2

The Gospel of Leukemia

The day my older brother and sister took me to see the doctor was the ultimate doomsday for me. I was expecting good results from the comprehensive blood work because the nurse had taken so many vials of blood from me.

I was very wrong. The doctor openly discussed with both of them that what I had was not just acute anemia. It was more (there's that word again) fatal, and I would have to be hospitalized at once. My illness could not wait. In fact, I needed a massive blood transfusion immediately.

The doctor called my illness "acute lymphocytic leukemia." I had no clue what was going on. I mean, I was fifteen years old. Whatever it meant, my sister started crying, and my brother shook his head.

I thought my illness was simply due to chronic monthly loss of blood and poor nutrition. But no, it was far more serious. I said to myself, "I am going to die." It was so terrible.

My brother and sister were speechless and told the doctor we would have a family conference to decide what to do with me. Of course they couldn't decide right in that moment.

They had barely scraped the money together to pay for the blood test and consultation, let alone to bring me to the hospital emergency room. The doctor had dropped atomic bombs on us—health bombs and financial bombs. It was horrendous.

The following day we all went home to bring the bad news to my mother and father. My father was brave in accepting the news. Thank God he didn't try to set up a lottery to see what date I would die on. That would have been kind of depressing.

I saw my mother cry. I could sense that she didn't want lose another child so young. My younger brother, Mario, had died when he was only seven years old. He died in the arms of my mother. I know now that his illness could have been cured if we had the money for doctors and medicine. Mario was three years younger than me, and he died of diphtheria.

In this day and age the disease is curable with antibiotics like penicillin. How could this have transpired? Well, for one thing, going for a general checkup for simple illnesses was not a usual practice for indigent people in the barrio, and that included my family.

Again—and I know I am not the second coming of Florence Nightingale—it is a lesson well learned for me now. God willing, I will do my best to always have the medical mission at my resort for as long as I live. No child of God should have to suffer like myself or my brother because of lack of money and preventive medicine.

Going back to my own predicament of having blood cancer

is a different story. I didn't know at that time that I could have the very same genetic blood disorder that my niece Sandy died of just two years before. (I will explain that whole scenario later in this book.)

Sandy's bleeding was mostly internal. My bleeding was mostly external, and it lasted for days on end. You might recall a story in the gospels about Jesus healing a woman with a blood disorder. For the grace of God, why do serious illnesses strike the same family? Is it the test of faith? Or is it in our DNA? DNA wasn't discovered until 1944. The human genome was not cracked until the summer of the Y2K. Understanding DNA is a relatively new phenomenon. Blood disorders are apparently as old as mankind. Don't get me started on how they used to bleed people with leaches in the Middle Ages.

And so, the family conference was indeed held between my father—whom you might know from that Kenny Rogers song "The Gambler"—my hysterical mother, my two older sisters, and my older brother. You know that TV show *House*? This wasn't *House*.

The decision was made to take me to a "faith healer." It is a decision frequently made by poor people in the barrio who don't watch the TV show *House*, and even if they do.

There was no way we could afford the hospital, the blood transfusion, the medicine, and all the comings and goings hospitalization entails. I mean, let's get real. If we could hardly afford to buy food, how could we afford all of those expenses?

At that moment, my mother cried so much. I know it was not because she would have to sell her precious Singer sewing machine, but rather the thought of losing another child.

I mean, look at my family and the vanishing people—my brother Mario, my niece Sandy—what is this, the Bermuda Triangle?

I know my mother began praying for me. I would always see her at night in the dark on her knees with her hands up in the air. Then she would bow to the bamboo floor. She had faith and knew the right source to go to for a miracle.

A few days passed. The faith healer came and instructed my mother and father what herbal medicines they'd been to gather for me to take. He also told my parents about food supplements they would have to feed me every day.
It was like, "Oh, go to the Afghani restaurant and get some fried leaves ..." This was going to cure me? Was I *Bambi* in the forest?

But faith healers and natural herbalists have their own methods, I suppose. I was just a little girl with a fatal illness. What were these concoctions anyway? Well, there were herbal roots and twigs of some rare trees that turn red when they are boiled. I am sure this has you bursting with confidence at this point.

I had to drink that mixture of roots and twigs every hour 24/7. There was raw egg yolk (like in the first Rocky movie) and a half-cooked liver, which I had to consume almost every day. The worst was the cod liver oil by tablespoonful. I endured it all, as I saw the sacrifices my parents were making to enable me to survive leukemia via eggs and twigs.

And roots—you can't forget the roots. Roots were good.

The news of my serious illness spread through the whole barrio. Every night people came to my deathbed to pray for me. We had a throng of visitors coming from miles away to pray for me to get well. Let's face it, they had to pray. I mean, who really believed I was going to get better by eating roots, twigs, berries, cod liver oil, and fried leaves from an Afghani restaurant? Not that we had an Afghani restaurant. We didn't. But you get the point. No one was like, "Oh, don't worry about the leukemia, honey, just drink some raw eggs and you'll be fine."

I just closed my eyes from time to time and asked God and His angels for a miracle. The angels were probably flying up to heaven and telling God, "There's this girl in the PI, and she has leukemia. They're giving her eggs and twigs and berries and stuff ... and God, well, you've gotta do something. You've gotta do something right now!" God created all the angels, and you can read about them in the Bible in Hebrews 1:1–4, Luke 20:34–36, Mathew 25:41, Revelation 5:11–12, Hebrews 1:6–7, and Acts 12:7–10

I guess I should throw in the fact that I was fifteen years old when I was struck down with leukemia, in case you forgot. And I was also raped during this very same year. Rape, leukemia, raw eggs, twigs, cod liver oil ... it never let up.

I was too tired to live and too scared to die. If it was my fate to die, I wished for it happen soon. I was so very tired of taking all those herbal medicines and seeing my mother and my whole family suffer with me. In all honesty, I didn't want to die, as my dreams would also vanish with me.

When it was very late at night and everyone was sleeping except me, I saw my mother praying the rosary and asking the Blessed Virgin Mary for divine intervention.

I realized then how precious I was to my mother, just as my son is precious to me. (I'll also get to that part of the story.)

Was I a part of God's perfection in my mother's life? She had been through so much.

My mother's cross was not only very heavy, but it was also really weighing her down. My illness wasn't leaving me. In fact, more complications began to appear from nowhere.

After a month of taking the herbal medication, my skin turned very yellow. The urine I excreted was dark orange. I was always nauseous and just could not eat anymore. I couldn't eat practically anything being offered to me. I was not getting better, and my condition was becoming worse and worse.

I thought, *Now I am **really** going to die.*

At that period in time, I resigned it all to my fate. I thought, So be it. *I will not go to school, and I will not become a photojournalist. I lost my star in the sky. My name will be erased forever.* I cried alone in silence. I wondered if my guardian angel was at my side.

Ever the gambler, my father (remember, he was a pseudo-shaman and medicine man) summoned the faith healer once again. When he came and saw me, he prayed, felt my pulse, and said to my parents that a miracle had just occurred. I

was cured of my blood disorder—the very same disorder the laboratory and the doctor called cancer of the blood. The disorder they called leukemia.
How could it be possible?

I was feeling worse and jaundiced beyond recognition, and he was saying I was cured.

The faith healer explained that because I was anemic and very weak, I was susceptible to any type of infection. He also said that because of the variety of herbal medication I had taken, my liver could no longer process my intake.

Looking back from the standpoint of 2011, I am thinking that the infection came from all the half-cooked liver, raw egg yolks, and other foods that were not properly processed or prepared.

The faith healer said to take me to a doctor for another evaluation. He also told my parents not to worry about my jaundice, as it was not a fatal disease. What he didn‘t tell them, or rather ask them, was, "Do you have insurance?"

There‘s a song from a film called Coal Miner‘s Daughter that goes like this: *"We were poor but we had love, that's the one thing daddy made sure of ... he worked hard to make a poor man's dollar ..."*

My mother‘s sadness went away. She was relieved, as if the heavy cross she had been carrying around was lifted off of her shoulders.

Matthew 11:28 reads, "Come to me all you that are weary and are carrying heavy burdens and I will give you rest."

Matthew 11:29 states, "Take my yoke upon you and learn from me; for I am gentle and humble in heart and you will find rest for your soul."
As I lay down that night, I thought of how my mother prayed to all the angels and the Virgin Mary. Maybe a miracle did occur on my behalf because of my mother's undying devotion.

Mother Mary is the mother of God. If you pray to her, maybe she will listen to you.

Luke 1:30 reads, "Do not be afraid, Mary, for you have found favor with God."

A mother's prayer to the Lord for the sake of her child is priceless. My mother was my angel during this difficult time, and her prayers might have been answered by God through the Virgin Mary. I don't know how else I can explain my miraculous recovery from leukemia.

— — —

There was another family conference waiting to be held, and this time my parents asked my married oldest sister to help out with expenses of bringing me to a doctor in Manila.

Since my sister and her husband didn't have any money either, they sold their cow to come up with the money, and in return my father told her she could have few more square meters added to their lot. (My oldest sister and her family lived adjacent to us.) They agreed to my father's astute proposition and sold their cow so we could afford the trip to Manila and various other expenses.

It was the beginning of rainy season, and the trip would be detrimental to my already weakened body, so they hired a private Jeep to take me to my other sister's house which was in Manila. Before the modern infrastructure development in the area, there was always flooding and pools of stagnant water everywhere. It was very difficult to make a trip to the emergency hospital. My sister still had to work and could not afford absences. Her income was vital to making ends meet. But God was still in control, along with His angels. The Bible tells us that every hair on our very heads is numbered and that God knows when even a sparrow falls. How much more valuable are you?

Luckily there was a doctor who had a private practice near my sister's house. The doctor made the diagnosis without even taking blood sample. She (the female doctor) said what I had was highly contagious and that I should be isolated. There was no isolation in the one-bedroom house, of course.

My treatment was very painful—an intramuscular injection in my butt every day with a very long needle. The syringe was filled with very thick vitamin K. Every time I got the injection, I cried out very loudly. As I am writing this, I am reminded of my past suffering. How did I endure all of it?

In the meantime, the H-fever epidemic became rampant in Manila. Wouldn't you know it, I became one of victims of the virus. Of course, we did not know about it. My sister thought that my fever was from my existing infection. Whatever ...

When my brother came to visit me, I was convulsive with high fever. I was also bleeding heavily, and blood was all over my mattress and my blanket. When my sister came home from work shortly thereafter, they called an ambulance and I was brought to the emergency room at Philippine General Hospital. I went through a battery of medical tests and further lab work. They also called in a gynecologist examine me. I found out later on what had happened to me, and it was very painful. It made a scar in my soul so deep that only the good Lord was able to heal it.

I had been raped, even while near death. (There‘s no need to comment here.)

After all the testing was done, I was transferred to a ward with about sixty patients. The hospital was overcrowded with patients, as it was the hospital for all indigent sick people from all over the country.

The doctors didn‘t have any choice but to confine all the patients to the hospital ward regardless of what kind of disease that person might have had. So I was thrown into a sea of dying patients. Well, I was one of them anyway. Again, who am I to complain? The Lord had brought me this far.

I endured pain and loneliness, as I did not have daily visits from my relatives or my parents. It was just too far and too expensive to come and visit me. But they had again proved their love for me. Oh, how it must have pained them to have been away from me at that time.
They were so close to finding a complete cure for me. We had come so far together as a family, and now I was out of touch in a physical sense. I bet they were praying for me, however, harder than ever.

I endured so much pain from all the interns practicing on my veins so they could learn to draw blood the proper way. The doctors actually made me a "case study." (It was like, "Oh and don't forget *not* to let Julie die for your medical school homework!") I stayed at the hospital until they decided it was time for me to be released.

I was very thankful that I was cured of infectious hepatitis, hemorrhagic fever, and a deadly form of leukemia.

Surprisingly, the doctors there did not find a trace of cancer. They found that I was very anemic. I had blood transfusions but no cancer. I became a grateful guinea pig.

Once again, I wish to say that my mother had a lot to do with my recovery. She was my angel. She had asked God to spare my life so I could go on with my dream.

John 14:13–14 reads, "Whatever you ask in My name, this I will do, that the Father may be glorified in the Son. If you ask me anything in My name, I will do it."

Matthew 10:22 states, "He that endures to the end shall be saved."

Psalm 27:14 reads, "Wait on the Lord: be of good courage, and He shall strengthen thy heart: wait I say, on the Lord."

During this chapter of my life, I realized that God does not intend to harm us. If you can see through your suffering, you will realize that it is also your opportunity for great joy.

We are not born to be miserable. Rather, we are born to experience life. Life is full of bumpy roads and potholes. It is up to us to find solace and comfort, knowing there is God and He is the Light at the end of our tunnel.

"All the world is full of suffering. It is also full of recovering."

—Helen Keller

Chapter 3

Coming to America the First Time

To this date, there are about 102 million people in the Philippines. The country is ranked as the twelfth most densely populated in the world. Friendship, commitment, and bonding in families are the common traits of Filipinos. You will find no truer friends once you befriend one of them. You will also be amazed at the commitment and sacrifices they are willing to endure for the sake of their loved ones.

If you ask them to walk a mile, they will walk a hundred miles with you. I say this because my US citizenship did not rob me of my Filipino identity. I do all of the above and also witness my *kababayan* (fellow immigrants) doing the same.

The Philippines is overburdened by a large national debt dating back to the Marcos years of plunder and extravagant lifestyles (Imelda and her three thousand pairs of shoes), leaving tens of millions of people in poverty.

The country's economy has always been kept afloat by the remittance of huge overseas workforce. Considered the new heroes, the Filipinos abroad send into the country billion of dollars, thereby saving the Philippines from total economic collapse.

I myself helped my family avoid financial hardship by being able to immigrate to the United States twice, working diligently, and saving money.

Luke 1:37 says, "For nothing is impossible with God."

I considered both of my entries to the United States miracles of God in my life. You might ask, "Why are they miracles?" They are indeed.

First of all, my parents were very poor. They could not afford to send me to school or buy my siblings basic necessities. How could they afford to send me to the United States? They could not afford bus fare to Manila. How could they afford an airplane ticket for me to go halfway around the world?

Consider the huge population of the Philippines. Most of them would love to trade places with me. I've been asked many times how on earth I managed to come to the United States not once but twice.

They could be highly educated or rich and famous, but only those who are petitioned by their next of kin or are legitimate tourists are able to obtain US visas. I heard through the grapevine one reason why. Four out of five Filipinos do not go back to the Philippines. They find that America is truly a great country and a land of opportunities. There's no going back till they make their goal of comfortable retirement, so most of them stay longer than they are supposed to.

Ask any Filipinos what they do for a living and they will tell you they are either nurses or they work two jobs. They live on the salary they make on the first job and send or save the money that comes from the second job.

I can attest to the fact because that is how I did it. I worked three jobs—two regular eight-hour jobs and side work on weekends.

This is the story of how I came to the United States for the first time. After my recoveries from various fatal illnesses, I believed there were still miracles waiting for me. I believe God created an opportunity for me to save my family from financial hardship.

The opportunity came when I heard there was someone from Manila looking for a suitable nanny-governess to three young daughters of a couple of doctors residing in the United States.

After hearing the news, I immediately asked my mother and my father's permission to apply for the position. My mother granted my wish immediately. I had a hard time convincing my father. He looked at the markings in the palm of my hands and shook his head. In my mind I asked, *Are you reading and predicting my future in a foreign land?* I never learned his thoughts at that moment in time, but I sensed he was worried about me. He even kidded that even if he built the biggest kite to ride on he would never be able to visit with me. It was a very touching statement of love, and I will never forget those words.

After much prodding and convincing from my mother and me, my father eventually agreed, saying, "I cannot give you wealth, but I can give you your wish to be free."

It was not my wish to leave, but it is a great calling to be able have a job and presumably find the way out of bleak future for all of us. Love alone was not enough to make me happy—not when there was a dream waiting to manifest and all I had to do was make the sacrifice to leave my family, work hard, and save money.

The arrangement was made between the recruiter and my parents. Under the agreement, the new employers, who were both doctors in New York City at the time, were to obtain proper documentation for me to work for them, pay my airfare to the United States, and pay me $100 monthly. My obligation was to take care of their three daughters ages seven, four, and three for five years.

I was only eighteen years old at that time. I was very naive and not knowledgeable of my rights. I say that because I just went along and never asked any questions.

I was required to have my training period at my employer's parents' house in Manila. In that house lived six adults and two children, boys ages six and four years.

While on training, the family paid me forty pesos a month, which was the equivalent of less than four dollars during that time.

I can tell you that my training was very rigorous. I trained not only to be a nanny-governess but also as a housekeeper. The family taught me how to use all modern appliances and also taught me how to cook. Our cooking in the barrio is much simpler. We either steam, boil, or broil, with no other ingredients but salt and pepper.

I worked from 5:00 a.m. to 7:00 p.m. seven days a week. My job consisted of cleaning the huge house manually. I was on my knees waxing the floors and buffing them shiny with coconut husk. This was done very early in the morning before I served them breakfast.

My typical days for months was around the clock waiting to serve three meals, clean, and retreat to the hardwood floor to rest and sleep for the night.

I fought my loneliness and surrendered to my self-pity in the darkness of midnight.

Tears marked my pillows in the morning, but I never thought to give up. I had my dreams, and they would materialize in God's time.

My temporary employers allotted me time to attend church. I am Catholic, and I attended mass every Sunday. I prayed to God to grant my wish sooner than later, as my days were getting longer and my nights seemed shorter.

It was a hardcore practice of being away from my family for months at a time. I could not even visit with my older sister, who lived only twenty blocks away. I was making such a small amount of money that I couldn't spend the money on bus fare to the province. I preferred for my mother and my younger sister come to see me, which they did occasionally in eight months. I gave them money each time.

They had to pay back the money they borrowed to fund each visit. Manila is a ten-hour round trip from my barrio, and it was not comfortable travel. First they had to take the overcrowded Jeep and then the bus, and then they had to either take a tricycle or another Jeep to go to where I lived. We always had a joyful visit, and then we would sadly say our good-byes. We hugged and kissed enough to last till their next visit.

In those days, I always felt like a prisoner of my dreams. I felt I would never be free until my dreams came to fruition. Dreams should be free. They should not be out of touch with reality.

I believe that I am not in this earth to be just a living, breathing thing. I believe God designed a beautiful, interesting life for me.

At that stage in my life, I felt like a cocoon. There was a magnificent butterfly waiting to fly out to the world of beauty.

On my seventh month of waiting, good news arrived. I would be leaving for New York the following month, which was June. All my paperwork was submitted to the US embassy, and I was just waiting for the release of my visa. Again, I did not ask any questions about how it was obtained, and I never saw my passport.

I had mixed feelings about the great news. I was happy I was finally leaving, but also very sad I'd be so far away from my family. I would not see them for five years. My employers let me take few days vacation to be with my parents and siblings. I went home all excited, knowing the door of opportunity just had swung open for me.

Just imagine—I was the first person from the whole barrio and even the whole town to go to America during that time. It was like getting lottery ticket with winning numbers. After my family reunion, I went back to Manila.

Usually when someone is going on a trip, a person needs to get his or her travel clothes ready. No, not shoeless Julie.

That time it was "no-suitcase Julie." I did not have much clothing to pack. I only had bare necessities, and there was no need for me to bring my own, as I would be a traveling companion to my employer's sister-in-law.

I always use that storyline nowadays when I tell stories of my humble beginnings. I say, "When I came to the United States, I did not even have a suitcase. Now, I have a walk-in closet full of designer clothes and shoes." How my luck changed is really a blessing from God.

My departure day came very fast. My family came—all of them. They hired a Jeep to bring everyone to the airport to see me for the last time. I cried, my mother and father cried—everybody cried.

Everyone was supposed to be happy, but not my family. Everyone was sad.

My first departure was very sentimental, and recalling it makes me realize the value of kinship and the lesson, "There's no place like home." Home is where the heart is, and going to an unknown destination for the first time took all my courage. I was afraid, but I had to go search for the "pot of gold."

The plane ride was exhausting. Our port of entry was Hawaii. I was not interviewed by immigration officials. I heard my employer‘s sister-in-law say I didn‘t speak the English language, so she did the talking and answering for me.

I never saw or even handled my passport, and it was kept from me until I left my employers five years later. I needed my passport to go home. It‘s sad but true, but on my third year with the family, I discovered I was one of the undocumented aliens living in the United States at that time. I didn‘t know I was only given one-month tourist visa as a "traveling companion" to my employer‘s sister-in-law.

After I arrived in the United States, my employers, who lived in New York City at the time, moved to Brooklyn, and after a year, they moved to Chambersburg, Pennsylvania. All those moves made me untraceable by Immigration and Naturalization Services.

I learned later on that I could not obtain a green card or immigration status because they let my visa expire without applying for the proper work permit for me to be able to stay in the United States permanently, all of which put me in sad situation. Not having proper documentation did not allow me to obtain a driver‘s license. My going out was left to the mercy of my neighbor and friend Carol or the girls‘ piano teacher when I cleaned her house.

Imagine being in the same environment doing the same thing religiously seven days a week with no meaningful activities that can alleviate homesickness. My loneliness was killing me. I tried everything possible to cure my boredom. I learned how to sew, I did embroidery, and I wrote letters and poems. I read many books, including my employer‘s

Physician's Desk Reference and New England Journal of Medicine, all of which later on I realized I benefited tremendously from, but I also used it to hurt myself.

From learning how to sew, I found my hidden skill. From writing letters and poems, I discovered my passion. From reading different books and journals, I educated myself in many aspects of science, medicine, and psychology.

Somehow during that time, I lost my focus on my dreams. I gave up on my willingness to accept my situation. I was hurting inside, and my vision of tomorrow was not visible anymore.

I continued to pray to God to give me back my hope, but my loneliness clouded my reasoning, so I decided to end my life to suffer no more. One day when the family left me, I took a massive dose of sleeping pills from the physician's sample boxes. I know it was an amount enough to make me sleep and rest forever. But God, again, intervened and did not let me die.

I woke up being worked on by the doctors trying everything humanly possible to make me survive. They induced vomiting to empty my stomach of the remaining sleeping pills. I know that they did not bring me to the hospital to avoid the embarrassment of being found out that they were employing an undocumented alien or a possible investigation as to why I tried to commit suicide.

The doctors left me in my room when they thought they had saved my life, only to find later on when they checked me again that I had slashed my left wrist with a blade and was bleeding on top of a waste can. Even when I was extremely confused and drowsy, I was thoughtful enough not to leave a mess.

There must have been an angel and a devil fighting over me at that time. I was still trying to be thoughtful in my hour of grief and disillusionment.

Again, the doctors were frantic to save me and, thank God, they were both in the saving lives profession. My wound was superficial, as I was very weak and almost too incoherent to have inflicted deep wounds. They cleaned, medicated, and bandaged my wrist.

My employers realized the seriousness of my suicidal tendencies, and they were afraid I would try it again. They asked me if I would like to go away, and they called my first cousin living in New York City. At that time my cousin was living with a nice family who would become my second employer seven years later. They had two young children and needed a part-time babysitter.

I kissed, hugged, and said good-bye to the family I had learned to love for three years.

They put me on a Greyhound bus to New York City and, six hours later, I was back at my first destination—the city that never sleeps.

The Kasilags welcomed me with open arms. I became a part of the family and not as their babysitter-housekeeper. They loved to go out on family picnics and usually traveled on weekends, and I was always invited to come. I made friends with people they knew and began to have a social life. It was a social life cut short because my former employers started calling me to come back to their home. They even had the three girls talk to me. They said they missed me so terribly, cried, and begged me to come home. The doctors also said they would double my salary from $100 to $200 and they would give me days off. They also said they would get a lawyer to fix my visa. That was a promise that never became a reality, because either the lawyer they hired was incompetent or it was not feasible.

Because I knew I would not be able to find a job in New York , I decided to go back to Chambersburg and fully braced myself that I would face the same predicament of being without friends and alone most of the time. I resolved to fight and be strong. I devotedly went to church every Sunday and learned to read the Bible when sadness struck me. The thought of being with God made me strong every day until it was time for me to go back home.

I planned my future and saved all my earnings from cleaning my friend Carol's apartment, the children's piano teacher's house, and my meager salary from my employer.

My plan was to continue my education when I go back to the Philippines. To do that, I had to have steady income. I wrote my older brother to find me a business that would allow me to have time to go to school. We sent letters back and forth.

He told me that he found a business with great income potential and to send him the money for capitalization. He also told me not to tell anyone, including my parents, about it. I complied with his request. I withdrew all the money I saved in the bank and sent it without second thought that the decision would bring a major catastrophic effect to my life.

Chapter 4

The Goodness of the Lord

The goodness of the Lord is the light I will follow.

You might be asking right at this very moment, “Julie, how did you survive such poverty, multiple rapes, leukemia, and emigrating from your country?” As for the latter, I can see that Jesus Christ Himself was driven out of many places and was usually “on the road again,” like in that catchy Willie Nelson song.

I would point to a verse of Scripture about the narrow road that leads to eternal life and the wide path that leads to destruction. Some people have heard of the narrow road and seeking the narrow gate. Some wonder how to find it or if they will ever be worthy enough to find it. Others simply don‘t care about any road—the narrow or the wide.

If you want to know what my magic formula is, I can tell you that there isn‘t one. What I can tell you is that God has filtered from my life what is useless. Discouragement is one of those things. Discouragement can break you. Fear can paralyze you for sure, but true brokenness can cause you to wind up in the wrong place. Sins always mislead us.

I will not confuse my soul and end up in hell. That's why Jesus came to this terrestrial plane: to save the lost from hell. Pastor John MacArthur and others, like Charles Stanley have hit on this theme, along with Paul Washer.

It is the inescapable question. Will you avoid hell and go to heaven? And if you get there, why will Jesus have already told so many, "I never knew you ..." like they're pounding on the door to Noah's ark as the rains began to fall, starting the Great Flood?

If you don't know the following verses by heart, then you really should. I am not some Bible thumper, but we should all have at least a few key verses memorized.

Matthew 7:13–14 reads, "Enter by the narrow gate; for wide is the gate and broad is the way that leads to destruction, and there are many who go in by it. Because narrow is the gate and difficult is the way which leads to life, and there are few who find it."

Here are some of my other cornerstone verses.

Matthew 6:33 reads, "Seek first His Kingdom and His righteousness and all these other things shall be added unto you."

Psalm 20:4 reads, "May He give you the desire of your heart and make all your plans succeed."

Second Corinthians 9:8 reads, "And God is able to give you more than you need, so that you will always have all you need for yourselves and more than enough for every good cause."

Matthew 7:7 reads, "Ask and it will be given to you, seek and you will find; knock and the door will be opened to you." Psalm 20:4 reads, "May He give you the desire of your heart and make all your plans succeed."

Proverbs 3:5 reads, "Trust in the Lord with all your heart and lean not on your own understanding; in all your ways acknowledge Him, and He will make your paths straight."

First Thessalonians 5:16 reads, "Be joyful always, pray continually; give thanks in all circumstances, for this is God's will for you in Christ Jesus."

Galatians 5:22–23 reads, "But the fruit of the Spirit is love, joy, peace, forbearance, kindness, goodness, faithfulness, gentleness and self-control. Against such things there is no law."

While it is true that human beings are given free will to make right or wrong moral choices, it is our duty to seek God's will for our own lives. If the words of Jesus remain in our hearts and are not further erased from society, then we can work from a strong foundation. I believe if we stick close to God's Word, then we will be blessed.

Thus far I feel blessed. The door of opportunity has been opening for me. I'm receiving grace and blessings from God, and my source of happiness is the fruit of my labor.

I previously mentioned the works I am able to carry out at my resort in the PI on my birthday. I would like to share a little bit more about them. I mention them only to praise the Lord for the goodness of His abundance.

God is surely good.

First, I donated to the church in my town. I was able to employ many people who needed jobs. I rebuilt a dilapidated multipurpose shed for indigent people and spent ten hours painting it myself.

I gave free entrance to my resort for more than two hundred youth, a church priest, and deacons.

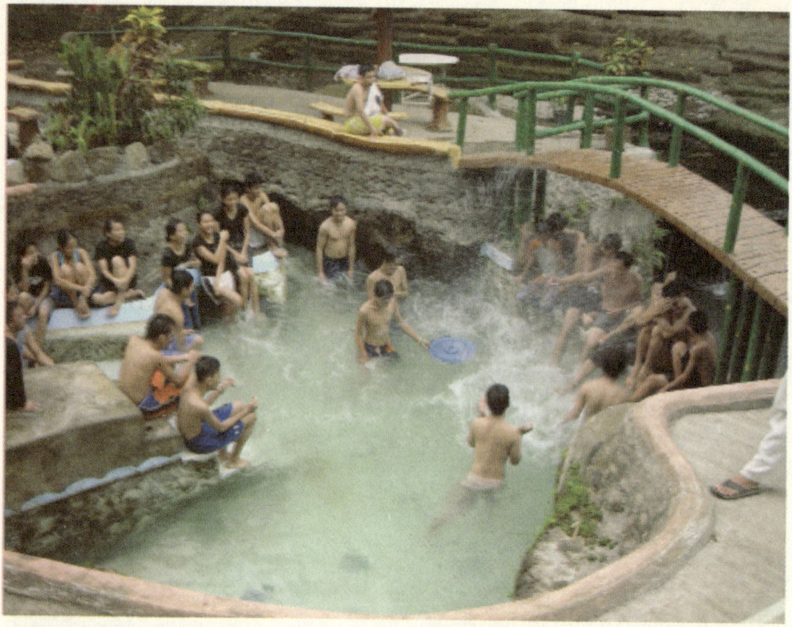

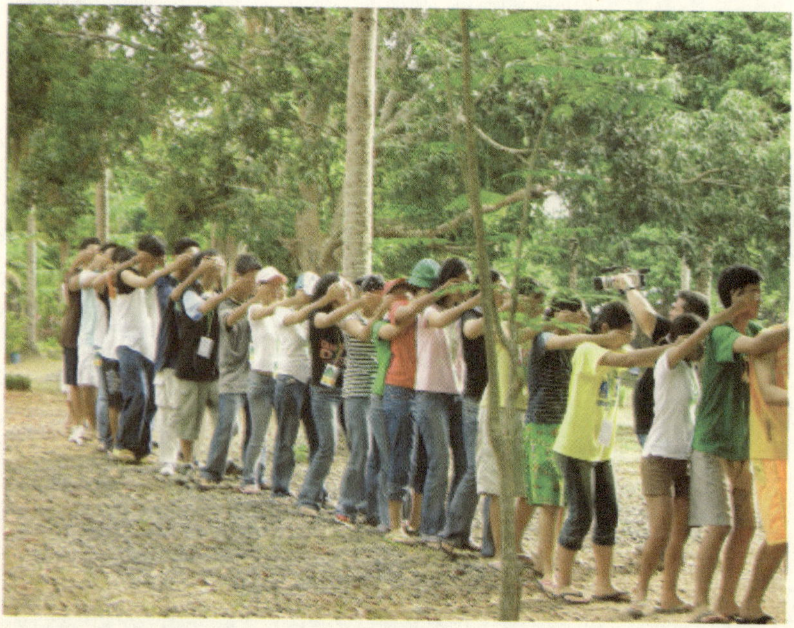

I also gave food and groceries to the poor people in the area.

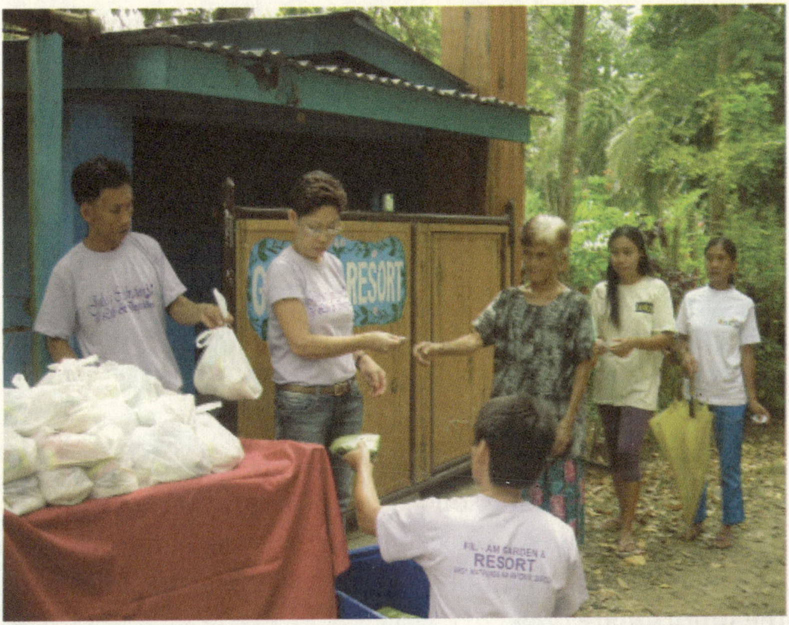

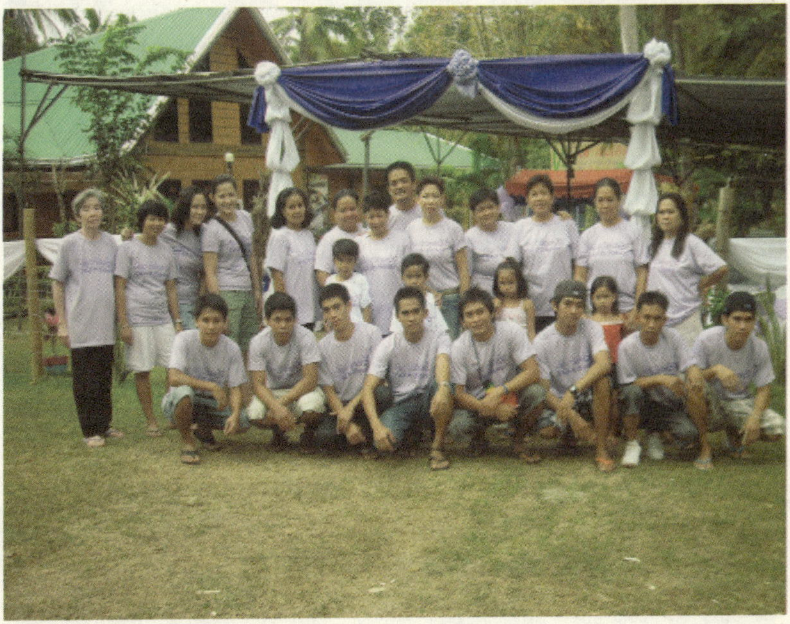

I gave gifts and bonuses to my resort crew, gave money and gifts to my brothers and sisters, and allotted dwelling property to my niece, my nephew, and my loyal carpenter.

The celebration went on all day, and the fireworks lit up the sky.

I felt God's presence all throughout that eventful day. I felt so close to Him. I felt as though I was seeing into the eyes of people who prayed for my health and for more success in this earthly life. It was the best birthday ever! It will be in my memory till the end of my days in this world.

So when I think on these things, the goodness of the Lord becomes the light that I follow. It took many years of waiting, but I am being given to (receiving) in the very same measure in which I gave. And more has been left over to share with the unfortunate ones.

Would you believe that I have recovered the land my father lost through his gambling? It is more land than I could have ever imagined, and it's in the same area. God is an expert at restoration, and all of the horrible things that have run over and through my body have found metaphorical cleansing in the mineral spring and pristine running water on my newly purchased land holdings. I buy each piece of land just a little bit at a time.

Make no mistake—I am patient, like Joseph was in Potiphar's jail. I bide my time for building a school here, an outdoor pavilion there, and a dorm to house twenty-four students. I ran an ad to bring Korean English- -as-a-Second-Language learners to my resort, and I found Anthony C. LoBaido somehow through that. He was busy at that time as a professor in South Korea training high-level members of the ROK Armed Forces, among other pursuits. It's like the

Great Wall of China; I am building it brick by brick. That's how life unfolds—bit by bit.

The good Lord gave me my heart's desires. I've always wanted to have a bed and breakfast, and now I have not only that, but a whole resort. It's my own piece of paradise where I can express my intuition and creativity.

I am able to enhance what God has created for me. He made it possible for me to plant five thousand mahogany trees and organize a garden to my heart's content and fulfillment. All of my plans are coming to fruition. I have been pushed and challenged. I have dared to dream and reach for an even higher level of spiritual life. I speak of a place where my own pain and suffering could be magnified and used to help others and thus bring healing to others and glory to the Lord.

I believe my values certainly played a major role in my present life. Had I not run with perseverance, I would not have all the blessings I'm enjoying these days. Had I not found God, I would be forever lost, like other souls who end up in the wrong places.

Love comes from the base of my heart. A great magnetic field five thousand times stronger than the brain comes from the base of my heart. I will decide from my heart with help from my brain, as "I'm ordering my future." I never thought I could indulge in my darkness and still have joy and dreams ... the difference is God!

— — —

I have many stories of love and kindness and God being my light as I travel a certain path. For example, I literally saved my little niece from a tragedy. She is my joy. She has lived with me and will celebrate her eighth birthday on April 24, 2011.

I also found a nine-year-old girl in my town who has multiple birth defects. Her parents were so poor and ignorant that they let their firstborn exist in a miserable state.

When I found her, she was not going to school, as she could not talk because she had a massive double cleft palate, which is a congenital fissure of the roof of the mouth. Imagine that. We take it for granted that we can talk. Shouldn't we use our words to glorify God?

How did I encounter this young girl? Well, a few years ago I was looking for a native bamboo cottage builder to use at my resort. I found the carpenter in town and at the same time found the little girl with birth defects in her mouth. I asked her parents about their daughter, and they told me her condition was beyond their control, as it was willed by God. They also didn't know how to go about asking for help. They were in a trap. They were resigned to fate. They were not out asking anyone about what to do and beating down the doors to find an answer.

I told them to bring her to me, as I would have (as previously mentioned in this text) a free medical-dental mission at the resort on my birthday. Her medical case was very complicated, and I went through many hoops and suffered from many broken promises before I was finally able to have her surgery done. She has been going to school since then.

I was very determined to help her so she could go to school. After few years of not giving up on her, her birth defect was finally operated on by the Mission of Mercy group of doctors from Washington DC. Praise be to God for His mercy!

You see how God works? He sent me to find the little girl. I became her angel. In our lives, we can actually become angels of sorts to someone we have not met.

Therefore, I continue to run toward the finish line of my dreams. As I run, I know the goodness of the Lord is the light I will follow.

Chapter 5

Money as God's Muscle

Long ago, the apostle Paul wrote "the love of money is the root of all evil." It's not the money in and of itself, which is simply a form of wealth to more easily facilitate barter. I mean, why not use chocolate bars instead of euros or British pounds or rands or won or baht or US dollars? I believe Paul was speaking about the love of worthless paper that is not liked to gold or silver. They are blips created out of thin air on a sleek computer screen by various central banks all around the world, but people are willing to live and even kill for it.

If the mysterious book of Revelation is to be believed, at some point in the future men will toss "sound money" like gold and silver into the streets as though it is worthless. One shivers to contemplate that scenario. But personally, I like to think of money as God's muscle. You know, to help pay for good works for others.
What do we hold, uphold, value, and treasure?

In Western civilization, it seems that God is no longer the measure of all things. Man and his money are the measure of all things. But let me tell you that neither man nor money is the measure of all things.

Letting money flow freely is the new eleventh commandment: "Do what thou wilt with thine money." Trillions of dollars flow across international boundaries daily. Consumerism is a new religion. The ethos of Charlemagne is long dead. Human identity has been shaped by nation, race, religion, gender, and family through the millennia. Yet, in the place of these things has arisen "Economic Man." Money often takes center stage. The Verve sings a song called *"Bittersweet Symphony"* in which the band claims, "You're a slave to money till you die."

We have seen where this new paradigm has led usregarding Wall Street, the big banks, and the global financial meltdown caused in part by synthetic derivatives. These complex financial schemes are so unruly that even the so-called elites don't understand them. You don't need a Harvard MBA to realize that printing up fake Monopoly money is not an answer and that debt is not wealth.

It is sweat and labor and hard work that matter most. Ideas like social credit are beginning to gain traction as people are waking up to the idea that modern man invented money through the Bank of England and then invented the ideas of credit, fractional reserve banking, and so forth. Since we as human beings invented this system, we can un-invent it. We don't have to build pyramids for the neo-pharaohs.

I mentioned buying up property on my land and how some of that land had natural springs with fresh water set upon these areas. Just as water flows like a river to the path of least resistance, money also flows. The Bible clearly says that God can offer blessings and take them away. God says not to trust in men and not to trust in riches. Again, God says to store our treasure in heaven.

So, too, do our lives and cognitive energies flow like a river. We have bad memories versus motivation, pain versus perseverance, and so forth. Please allow me to tell you that money can indeed be God‘s muscle to enable you to do the great things God wants to do for yourself, your family, children, strangers, and various others.

But money can also be a prison. Getting down to the brass tacks, since I have been through extreme financial difficulties and because of my unique challenges—no college education or other trade skills certificate I‘ve had to learn the hard way.

I am very thankful to the good Lord for my opportunity to come to United States. I found an employer in New Jersey who gave me a chance to work. They paid for my airfare. My contract with them was to stay and work for five years. The pay was not great, but I was able to find extra babysitting at night and also worked few hours at a neighborhood deli. It was very hard, because I was constantly juggling my time and trying to fit everything in my work schedule with my employers.

I believe you have to know what you want and be aggressive. You have to change and reinvent yourself like Rick Ankiel. He was a kid with one of the highest signing bonuses ever, was rookie of the year, was a left-handed pitcher ... and then he vanished from Major League Baseball for years, only to reemerge as a centerfielder with the best arm in all of baseball, making amazing catches, hitting a home run at Yankee Stadium, and other exploits. He actually hit twenty-five home runs in a single season.

Isn‘t that amazing?

Who would have thought Rick Ankiel could do what no other player in baseball history has done? Did I mention his rebuilt knee and elbow? Did I mention his father was put in prison for various federal charges on weapons and drug trafficking? Did I mention how no one believed in Rick Ankiel and how the baseball world turned their back on him? But the thing is, you have to believe that you can reinvent yourself. Again, I mention Joseph in Potiphar's jail. He went from prisoner to the ruler of all of Egypt.

As for my new bosses in New Jersey, no, they weren't *The Sopranos* of HBO fame, but they were very accommodating to me because they were not paying me even minimum wage. I was able to save most of my income. Eighty percent went to the bank and twenty percent went to support my parents. No friends and no going out was my motto. I did this for two years, and then I asked my employers if they would kindly let me out of my contract because I needed to make more money to secure my financial future. They understood and granted me my wish.

I continued to work in the deli, and then out of the blue I was recruited to work in a very upscale Italian-American restaurant. The owner took a liking in me and trained me to be their best waitress. I believe this was the Lord blessing me. I excelled in the area of customer service, which I developed following that experience. Every day I'd go to the bank with all the tips I made. I worked lunch and dinners for six days and a half day on Sundays and cleaned houses on the other half of the day.

This was not a balanced life, and I did not leave time for God on Sundays or any holy day. Perhaps I was just too caught up in the idea of work, work, work. Americans value work. They have longer workweeks compared to, let's say, Europeans. But you need to have a balance. Even God took a day off after creating the world. A day of rest can define your week. On the other hand, doctors, police, and firemen are needed to protect society, so working on the Sabbath day, whatever that might be, can be a noble thing for those kinds of positions. I tell you to work and work and do more work, but don't let work rule your life or ruin your health.

I've accumulated many business cards, mostly from men who wanted to give me another job, date me, or marry me. All the while I was laughing all the way to the bank and saving all my money. I mean, who wants to marry a waitress or a cleaning lady after a brief meeting? Get real ...

When someone who worked for a financial business tried to recruit me, I attended their seminar just to learn how to invest and how to grow money wisely. The Bible tells us to be wise stewards of our finances. This is important. There is no such thing as a free ride or a free lunch. In this world, you pay as you go.

I shopped at dollar stores and accepted hand me downs from my female restaurant owner. It's funny today how people pay premium prices for clothes that have holes and rips in them.

As was the case of building the Great Wall of China being built brick by brick, in four years I had saved enough money to put a down payment on a house. But I eschewed that and, along with five girls, I rented a two-bedroom house. I know this might sound weird, but I slept on the kitchen floor all those nights during the five-roommate era because I had a dream and swore that I'd never be poor again.

In fact, I felt that I would somehow be rich both ways—financially and spiritually. I don't mean to sound like super-pastor Joel Osteen. I am not talking about flying first class. I am talking about having enough to eat and some left over to give to the poor.

All the while I never forgot my parents and my siblings. I took care of my parents financially—especially during their illnesses. To be frank, I shouldered all of their expenses. "Honor thy mother and father." This commandment comes before "Thou shall not kill." Perhaps it is a worse sin to dishonor your parents than to commit murder in God's eyes.

When my sister's house which was in Manila burned down to the ground, I sent them money to build a new home. I risked sending the money in faith, and God multiplied my blessings anyway. Things kept going up and up for me.Some people would call it lucky. I just felt that the harder I worked, the luckier I became.

As you might well be aware, the restaurant business does not offer health benefits, so later on I decided to work in a nursing home as a nurse's aide from 7:00 a.m. to 3:00 p.m. I'd get up at 5:00 a.m. and take the bus at 6:00 a.m. to be at work at 7:00 a.m. By 4:00 p.m. I was at the restaurant working until 10:00 p.m. Was my body a temple at this time? Did I have a healthy balance? The answer is, of course, no. But sometimes you have to set aside a certain stage of your life to achieve such goals via extreme measures.

The interest on my money in the bank paid for my first car. I told everyone, "I'm as American as the blonde next door."

I loved my Chevrolet Cavalier, hot dogs, and apple pie. My life was not all that exciting because, as I said, I was driven by certain goals and fears, so I pursued every job I could to make money.

My second opportunity for investment was having the chance to work for a major department store. It had a phenomenal profit-sharing plan and a 401(k) plan. I took advantage of maximizing the pretax contributions. I selected an amount of ten percent and, after ten years of buying the stock and liquidating that stock within the company's plan, I amassed well over $100,000, which I rolled over to another broker when I left to develop my resort back in the Philippine Islands.

I don't have credit card fees. The bank pays me dividends, air miles or other benefits. I don't pay my broker because they give me free trades.

I don't have a lot of money, but my credit is beyond my wildest dreams.

When I went to Las Vegas a couple of years ago, I was able to buy a four-bedroom house in a week, and this was without income verification. I backed out of the deal because I became suspicious. My hunch was right—the housing bubble burst. I mention this because the whole housing debacle in which banks, regulators, and security traders created a horrible financial debacle which made a mockery of all I was trying to do.

How much you make, how much you keep, and how you use what God has given you are private workouts in God's gym, creating God's muscle for His use and His glory.

I also wish to mention that I did sewing and alterations during this time in my life. I did this for four years. Then I found a job at a photography store where I learned about cameras and many types of film. It was a fun job because I was able to study photography and film developing.

I was able to save enough money to just work one job and go to school three nights a week. I only was able to finish the equivalent of seventh grade in the PI, as you know by now, and I wanted to have a high school diploma through a GED program. I studied hard. I passed the tests and qualified to go to college, which was my dream.

First Corinthians 13:4–8 says:

> Love is very patient and kind, never jealous or envious, never boastful or proud, never haughty or selfish or rude. Love does not demand its own way. It is not irritable or touchy. It does not hold grudges and will hardly notice when others do it wrong. It is never glad about injustice but rejoices whenever truth wins out. If you love someone you will be loyal to him no matter what the cost. You will always believe in him no matter what the cost. You will always believe in him, always expect the best of him and always stand your ground in depending him.

All the special gifts and powers from God will someday come to an end, but love goes on forever.

This is the kind of love my mother has for my father. My father did so many wrong things in their relationship, but my mother stood by him through twelve children till the end of his time. My father passed away eight years ago, and my mother followed him the next year.

I am grateful to my mother for staying with my father through hardship and extreme poverty. If she would have left him on the eighth child, I wouldn't be here telling you my triumph over adversities. She was my angel during my leukemia and a role model of patience and perseverance. She was a good woman, a good wife, and a good mother. She earned her place in heaven.

What I witnessed in my parents' marriage, the difficulties of raising children, and what cruel and unfair men do to women made me totally not interested in any men at all.

I thought I would never fall in love. I thought I would never find someone who could meet my expectations. My expectations from men are simple: do not treat me as an object of desire. My horrendous experiences with men left me traumatized, and for a long time I had nightmares at night.

I was practically working three jobs—two full time and part time jobs on weekend. I worked at a nursing home from 7:00 a.m. to 3:00 p.m. Then I took the bus and worked at the restaurant from 4:00 p.m. till 10:00–11:00 p.m.
My third job was either housekeeping or odd and ends sewing and alterations.

I was really driven to earn money and save as much as I could. I promised myself I would never be poor again.

I also was sending my younger sister to college and supporting my parents financially at that time.

Of course, when you are a fairly attractive female and you work in a restaurant environment, you get propositioned by many men.

I made up my mind that no man, regardless how persuasive he was at the time, would ever get to sabotage my plan to get ahead in life. For me, men were just interested in my body, and just the thought of going out on a date gave me chills.

So I continued to work at the same restaurant for three years. I developed really nice clientele, and some of them became my friends. One of them, a man named Eddie, was always persistent about asking me to go out on a date. Of course, I said I couldn‘t. I told him I was too busy or I had somewhere to go. I‘m quite sure women swooned over him. He is tall, handsome, and rich.

Anyway, I gave myself a deadline. I said to myself, *If he does not give up in another three months, I'll go out with him.*

On the second month of my self-imposed deadline, he told me he was going to Florida and would be away for a month. He asked me to wait for him, meaning that I shouldn‘t go out with anybody while he was in Florida. I finally gave him my home number and waited for his call.

Can you believe that? I was actually going to wait for a man to call me and go out on a date.

In the meantime, I made myself busier. I bought myself a sewing machine and began accepting minor clothing alteration work. Most of the time my sewing work came from the owner of the Italian restaurant where I worked. As I was only using a very low coffee table, I needed a real sewing machine table.

I didn't know where I could buy one, and since my roommate knew my need, she recommended for me to see the man who always bought takeout food at the Chinese restaurant where she worked. She told me he worked at a bedding and furniture store few blocks from the house we were renting.

And so I did.

It was the day I will remember for the rest of my life. I found what I was not looking for—the man who would change my perception of men. He was the man who would become my tower of strength and Rock of Gibraltar.

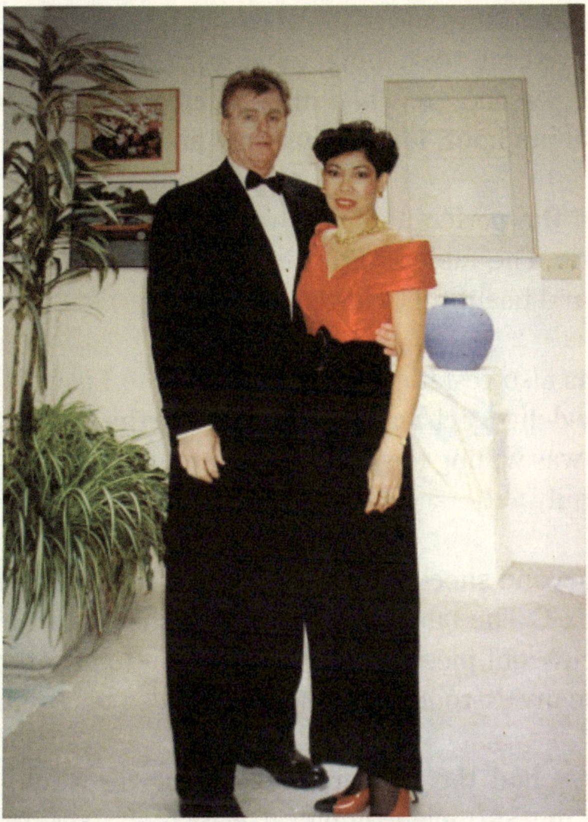

The store was huge. Inventories of beds and other odd and ends furniture were everywhere. I was welcome by a very distinguished gentleman with grayish hair. I never had any idea that he would be the man who later on I will call my PGG (perfect gift from God). I was not impressed by his looks. He was wearing what seemed to be an old-fashioned polyester navy suit. He was so fair skinned and so Irish looking—definitely not my idea of a good-looking guy.

Anyway, I shyly introduced myself, and he told me his name was Lou and he managed the store. He showed me around and was extremely attentive and friendly. I was very specific about what I needed. The table had to be small, preferably triangular, so it would fit in the corner area of my apartment. He showed me everything, including the closed-out pieces in their warehouse. Then after poking and picking for at least half an hour, I finally had my "aha moment."

I found the perfect table. It was so perfect that I actually kissed it. The table is French Provincial style and just so lovely and beautiful to have.

Lou was also ecstatic I found my table, so I asked the price and the delivery charge. I was expecting the cost to be above what I was willing to spend, but lo and behold, Lou told me it was only $10.

I was beyond shocked, and I said, "No way. It can't be. Are you sure?" The table looked very expensive, but he said it was a closeout piece and he was giving it to me at that price because my ex-roommate, Edith, was also his friend.

Then we had the delivery discussion. He would have to charge me $30 even though it was a very short distance, which I thought was ridiculous, so I told him "I will pay you the $10 and I will just put the table over my head and walk home since I live only three blocks away."

I told him that I was so used to doing that because when I was in the Philippines, I put the firewood I gathered for cooking over my head to carry it. I said, "It will not embarrass me, as doing it will save me $30."

Well, he took my $10, gave me my receipt, got a screwdriver, and began dismantling the table.

I didn't know what the heck he was doing until all the legs were separated and he started loading it to his car. The last piece that went in was the tabletop. It left just enough room for me to wiggle in and for him to drive three blocks to where I live.

I was shocked and speechless, but went along anyway. I just let a stranger decide for me. How did that happen? I didn't like it, but I couldn't say no. His action made my heart smile.

A few minutes later we arrived at my apartment, and he put the table together quickly. While I was serving Lou a refreshment. It was a surprise call from Eddie. He was back from Florida, and he was collecting on my promise to go out with him. He asked me if he could come over, since he was only across the street.

I said to myself, "Wow! This is really exciting." But then I looked at Lou just opposite me, and I had a sudden change of mind about what I was hoping to do when Eddie came back to go out on a date.

I sighed deeply and told him, "I'm really sorry but we can't go out anymore, as I am already committed to someone else."

I don't know what I was thinking when I said it, but Eddie was shocked and could not believe me. He asked me many questions, like, "How did this happen so quickly? How can you be committed right away when you just met the person ... and who is this man?"

This whole conversation was going on in front of Lou, and I sensed he was getting uncomfortable and getting ready to leave to go back to the store.

I told Eddie, “I am so sorry, but I cannot date two people at the same time.”

Here I was, telling the man I was waiting for that I was committed to someone I only met about an hour earlier. I already had a sense of loyalty to a man I barely knew. I didn‘t even know his status or if he had any romantic interest in me.

Anyway, I thanked Eddie for the call and said good-bye. I felt uncomfortable that Lou heard all of my conversation and thought I had just used him as my reason to refuse a date. Honestly, I knew my reason all along. I was not ready to go out on a date and would never be ready for the rest of my life.

Lou said good-bye and said, “I‘ll drop by one day to visit.” I said, “If you wish” just to be polite.

The idea of being with men or with a man alone scares the hell out of me. How could I ever start socializing with opposite sex?

Although I interacted with many men at the restaurant, I was always leery that they might have a hidden agenda. The trauma of having been violated cruelly left me very afraid of up close and personal relationships with any men.

At age thirty-two, I looked like I was only twenty-five and had many suitors, but they were just a bunch of no-good men to me.

A whole week passed by after I purchased my table. I was very happy with my table. Whenever I used it, I was reminded of how kind the manager of the store saved me the delivery charge and also how efficient he was at putting it together. In my own mind I thought, *There is still a nice guy left on this planet.*

I only worked at the nursing home Monday to Friday. At the restaurant, I worked only dinners on Saturdays and Sundays.

On Saturday mornings, I did all my errands, laundry, grocery shopping, cooking food for the whole week, among other things. On Sunday mornings, I usually had housekeeping jobs. It was my regular schedule, and I was quite happy with my financial situation. Despite my meager jobs, I was able to save money for my future.

One Saturday morning I was busy repainting my apartment, and I heard a loud knock on the door. I was perturbed, as I was working at a hectic pace and not expecting anyone, not even a mailman at that time.

I just continued painting, but there was more knocking, and it was really annoying me at that moment. I dropped everything, removed my gloves, and headed to the door. I was thinking that whomever was at the door, he or she was not going to get a very pleasant greeting—maybe even a four-letter word, which I am never comfortable saying.

I swung the door open, and there was Lou, coffee in one hand and a bag of doughnuts in the other. He was standing there with a big good-morning smile on his face. How could I ever get mad with that? I would be out of my mind if I did.

He handed me the goodies and simply said, "I was thinking of you this morning and thought perhaps you might like coffee and doughnuts." How did he know ? "Wow ... this is so very thoughtful of you," I said. After I said that, he left immediately to go to his work.

He did this a couple more times, sometimes missing me and then following me to the laundromat for my coffee and doughnut morning routine.

I had never been pursued in a such a respectful, caring way, and I didn't know what to think. All I knew was this: my trust for this man was growing by leaps and bounds. Heaven knows I was not falling in love. If there was such a word, it would be "falling in like." I still don't like a man in polyester suit. It is quite tacky.

I was not losing sleep as a sign of crazy feelings about this man. I just had many unanswered questions going through my mind, like, "Why is he doing these nice things for me? Why will he not tell me his intentions up front?"

Just when I gathered enough nerve to ask those questions, he asked me to come to the park one day when I was not working three jobs.

I smiled at his invitation. "Is there ever a day that I am not working?" I said to him.

"Well," he said, "here is my number. Call me if ever you have the time and we will have a nice picnic at the park nearby."

I told him I'd think about it. I thought about it for one day. I decided I would go, but I didn't call. A few days passed by and, because I was never idle, I completely forgot the invitation.

He must have been very anxious about the picnic idea, because he called when he thought it was convenient for me, and I said, "Yes, I will go." Away we went to Van Saun, a Bergen County Park ten minutes from my house.

Van Saun Park is beautiful and peaceful. It has matured trees, a running brook, and a huge pond. In the middle of the park is a small spring creek they call George Washington spring. There is a historic marker in place that claims George Washington and his armies rested and drank the water from that spring.

I immediately fell in love with the place and secretly made a wish that someday I would like to own a similar place.

Little did I know that my wish would be granted, and it is more beautiful on a grand scale, with mineral spring waterfalls, a spring creek lined with countless bamboo trees, mangoes, bananas, and bird of paradise plants.

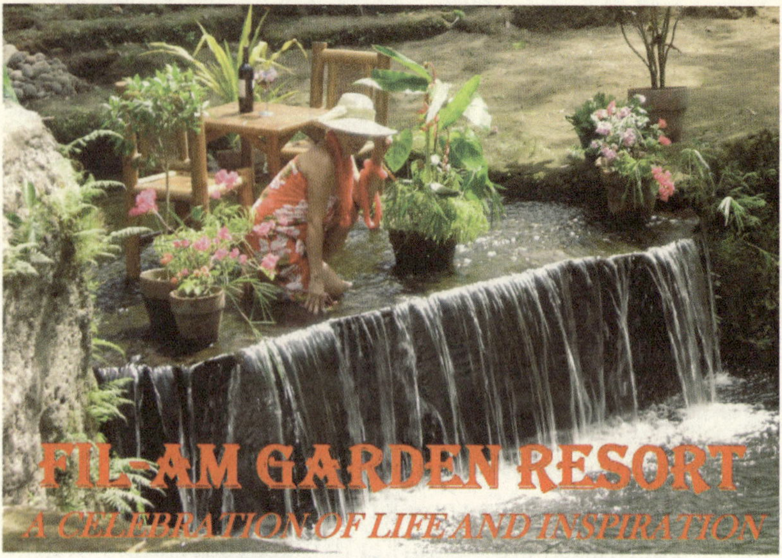
FIL-AM GARDEN RESORT
A CELEBRATION OF LIFE AND INSPIRATION

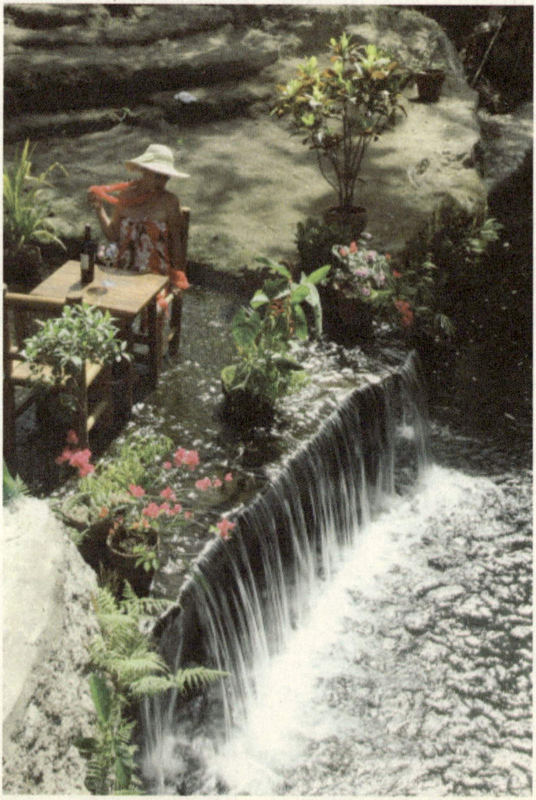

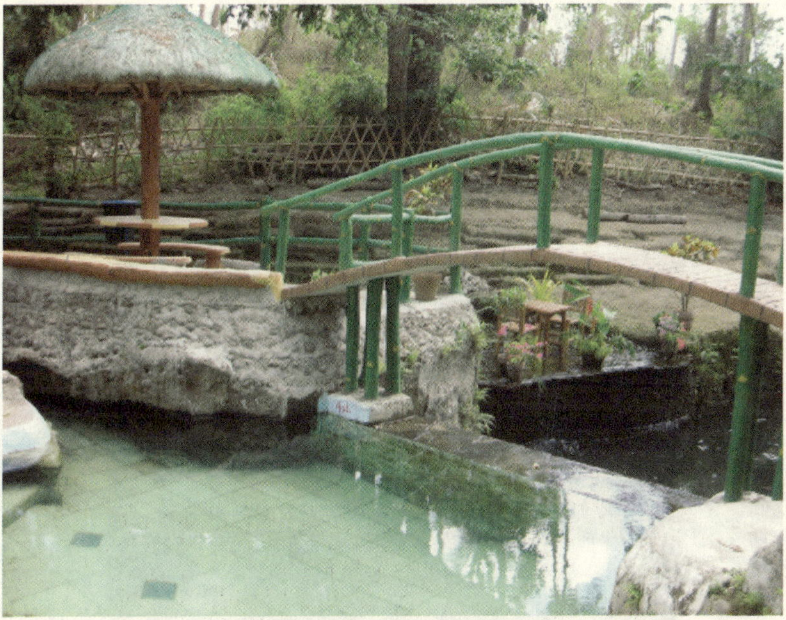

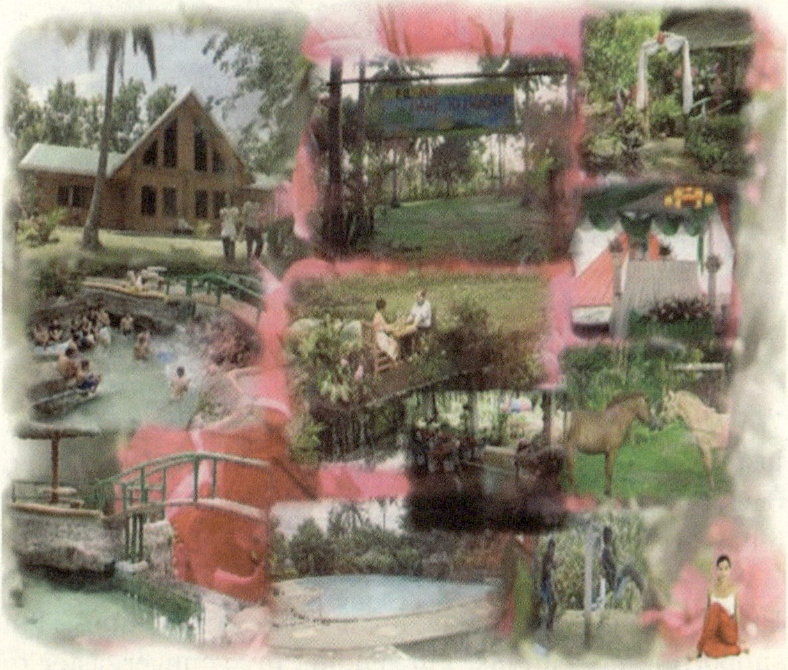

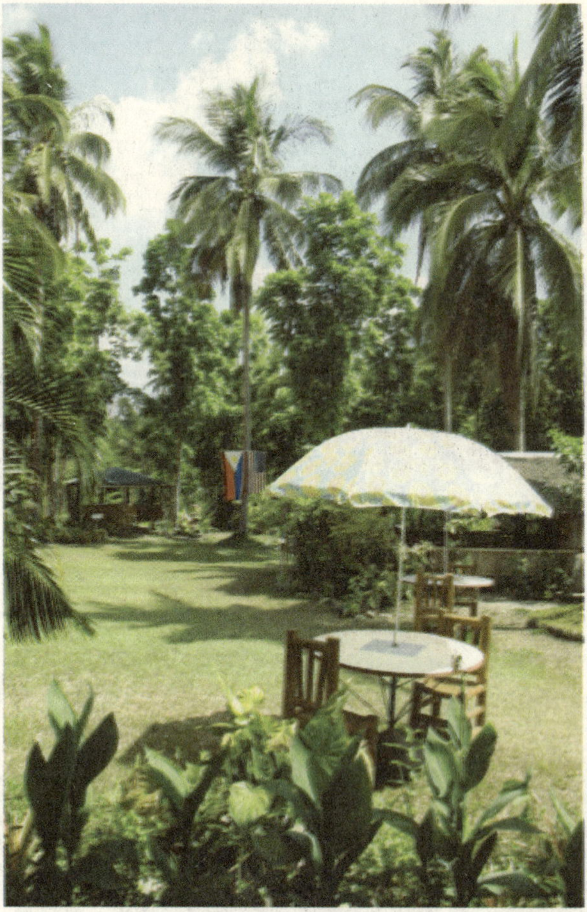

We chose a very cozy spot by a small wooden bridge and had our picnic there.

We were just quiet, just looking at each other, and then I just blurted out, “You know, this is not a date. I cannot go out on a date with anyone.” I just continued talking and telling him all the reasons why.

I said, “I have so many financial responsibilities. I‘m supporting my parents. I‘m sending my younger sister to college, and I'm saving money because I want to regain custody of my son that I gave up for adoption."

Nothing could stop me from all my plan, and I also said that if he fell in love with me, he would have to marry the rest of my family, and there were so many of us and we are all poor and needy.

After emptying what was in my heart, I started crying. He held my hand and said, "Don't worry. I'll be here for you. Where is your son? Where do they live?"

So I told him the rest of the story about my son's adoption. I told him how my friend Carol reneged on her promise that I would always be my son's mother and that she would never take him away from me completely.

I told Lou that they lived more than two hours away in South Jersey and I had only seen him once. Carol denied me further visits, as she claimed my son became confused about who his real mommy is. She told me that after my initial visit, my son started wetting his bed and she was afraid that he would develop serious psychological problems.

At that time I was crying and sobbing uncontrollably. He hugged me and said, "Give me their address and I will talk to Carol. This is not fair to you and your son."

He said his first opportunity was Sunday. We were at the park on Saturday at noon. He didn't even blink an eye. He was that serious. At that moment, I thought I fell in love.

I had never felt such compassion and so much caring from a man. I thought an angel had fallen from heaven at that moment. I thought, *I now have an ally. Can this be true?*

It was true. That Sunday he drove more than two hours to meet up with Carol. Lou found her working at Cape May County Hospital. He told her of his mission to help find a common ground for me to be able visit my son on a regular basis. Apparently Lou‘s visit disturbed Carol and her mother, who was living with her at the time.
They planned their exit from the area immediately and of course without my knowledge.

I placed countless calls, with no answer. In the end I just received messages that the number was no longer in service. I panicked and updated Lou about what was happening. He decided to go to where they lived. He found the house completely empty, and when he went to the hospital where Carol worked, he was told she was no longer there and they didn‘t know their where she went, as she did not leaved a forwarding address.

When Lou came back and delivered the bad news, he hugged me tenderly as I cried and cried for hours. When it rains in my life, true buckets of tears fall from the sky. This is one pain I don‘t know how to endure. It hurt so much not knowing where my son was and the thought that I may never see him again.

Lou visited me frequently during those times and even tried various measures to find them, but to no avail.

Lou and I grew closer to each other, and he learned so much about my life, my family, and most of all, my past suffering. He was always very compassionate and understood the sadness I was going through every day.

All I could do was hope and pray that someday I would see my son. It was prayer that would be answered fourteen years later.

Lou thought it would be best for me not to just dwell on my misery. He wanted me to go out and enjoy life. He convinced me to add sports to my hectic schedule. We both decided to start walking and running together, mostly on Sundays.

We trained together for various short running races. We also joined the New York Road Runners Club. Our relationship also grew, and he became my pillar of strength. He was always there when I needed a shoulder to cry on.

One day out of the blue a letter came from Harrisburg, Pennsylvania. The letterhead indicated it came from the office of an administrative judge. When I opened it, I discovered it was from Carol's brother, who was an assistant judge in Harrisburg.

The letter stated that I was not to continue to try to find Carol and my son, as they would deal with me accordingly, meaning they knew, that at that time, I didn't have proper documentation to stay and work in the United States.

It was another blow to my already sagging spirit. "How cruel can people be?" I asked myself. They had already reneged on their promises that I could see my son and I would always be known to him as his mother, but they were also blackmailing me. They also changed my son's birth name to Joey. To this day, I cannot bring myself to think and call him by any name other than Armand. He will always be my precious Armand till the day I die.

The judge also mentioned that all correspondence will go only through him. I prayed to God that such cruelty should not go unpunished. All I could do during those time was pray incessantly.

First Thessalonians 5:16 says, “Be joyful always, pray continually in all circumstances for this is God‘s will for you in Christ Jesus.”

Hebrews 12:1 says, “Let us run with perseverance the race marked out for us.”

A few more letters. Sometimes there was a good letter that contained some pictures of Armand and some school art he made. It did not appease my longing to see my son. I continue to beg Carol‘s brother to let me know where they lived, but my pleading fell on deaf ears.

Many years passed by, and I prayed and persevered. In one of my letters, I told the judge that even animals go crazy when their offspring get separated from them. How much more would it be true of a human being like me?
Again my pleading fell on deaf ears.

Finally, I let go and let God take care of my worries and suffering. I decided I could not go on well in life if I always thought of people who have hurt me. I had to learn to forgive all over again.

I am glad I did not give up on my life. As I look back through my years of hardship, failures, and heartaches, they are the components of what now makes my life beautiful and interesting.

When my life is full of doings, goings, and losing, it is also at the same time my learning, gaining, and receiving many blessings.

The bountiful life I have right now is because of my hard work. I learned so much from my father losing his property. I gained wisdom in life from the adversities I faced and survived. I reaped what I sowed, and God multiplied my blessings.

As I waited for the day when my son would come again into my life and we would be reunited, I busied myself more. I prepared myself to take courses at the nearby community college nearby, realizing my ultimate goal of finishing higher education by becoming a writer—a journalist.

But that dream did not materialize because I finally got married. Lou proposed to me in a very symbolic place at Cape Cod right on top of the Plymouth Rock. He said, "I am a pilgrim myself, and I have overcome similar obstacles to the people who came on the *Mayflower*."

He waited for me patiently for five years, and it was only fitting that that I said yes. It was the second week of October and a beautiful autumn morning.

We set the date of November 13 for the wedding, which is my son's birthday. We did not want a big wedding and only invited closed friends.

I bought pure white satin fabric and made my own wedding dress. It took me one week to make it, as I did not take vacation time. We prepared everything in a month, and we got married at the Hotel Thayer garden overlooking the

Hudson River. Hotel Thayer is the famous hotel at West Point Military Academy. Our wedding was beautifully officiated by West Point's appointed minister, Reverend Gehan.

Before the wedding, the minister asked to interview us. He asked us many questions. One of the questions he asked me was, "How do you know this man is the right person, and how do you know that your marriage is going to work?"

My answer surprised him. I said, "I consider Lou my perfect gift from God and whatever is in the box is mine. Love is not what I am expecting to get but what I am expecting to give, which is everything." A famous actress may have said that too, but I said it not knowing it was a famous quotation by somebody else.

I knew in my heart that when I got married, it would be forever. I have never known any man intimately other than Lou. I will never be comfortable with anybody else but Lou. Since I met him, he has been my knight in shining armor and my pillar of strength. He is true to his promises. When he married me, he married my entire family. He loves everyone I love, and I am grateful for that.

Because of Lou's generous spirit, I was able to continue to support my parents and also help my siblings financially when needed.

We traveled to different places on Sundays. We joined the New York Road Runners Club and ran races at Central Park. We did joyful things like picnicking in the park and visited many points of interest. Lou knows the passions of my heart are cooking and gardening, so he always finds great restaurants and botanical gardens.

I finally found what was missing in my life. When I found Lou, I found my happiness.

Being married and having a super sales-oriented retail career took too much time, and I just could not juggle both effectively, so I deferred going to college.

I concentrated on building my personal business both in the department store and back in the PI, and in no time I gained the store's recognition. I grew my sales upward and was a Pacesetter seven years in a row. I was a vested customer service all star. I was even invited to give a personal seminar on "How to Grow your Business" at our flagship store and also at the opening of another store as the company grew in our area. Can you imagine that?

Because I was a customer service board member, I was able to do a lot of volunteer work representing my company. My most enjoyable moment was the United Way's yearly campaign. We would go out and choose an agency to which we wanted to give time.

One day I was called to go down to human resources and, much to my surprise, the department manager handed me a huge Bergen County United Way calendar. When I flipped the page, I saw that they featured me in the month of August. The picture showed me singing to mentally challenged individuals in one of the agencies where we had visited and performed.

At the bottom of that picture in the calendar is the quotation, "Kindness is the only investment that never fails."

That is so very true. I say these things not to brag, but only to show God‘s goodness.

All the kindness I‘ve shown toward others has come back to me in so many ways.

Sometimes kindness is a powerful gift that can lift the spirit of a person having a challenging time. Sometimes kindness is just few words of encouragement or a simply a hug. You never know how even the smallest gesture of kindness can mean so much to others. Of course, this kind of decorum seems to be vanishing from Western societies.

I‘ve given so much to so many because I know what I needed (and so often lacked and went without) during the times of my sorrow—rape I, rape II, leukemia, two years at the garbage dump at Subic Bay in the PI. It comes so naturally for me in my everyday life to give hugs because I know that maybe that particular person is having an uphill battle in his or her personal life on that very day. God doesn‘t have any other lights for this place. You are the salt of the earth and the light of the world. If you don‘t shine, it‘s going to be dark.

First John 4:7 reads, “Let us love one another, for love comes from God. Everyone who loves has been born of God and knows God.”

Matthew 5: 13–16 reads, –You are the salt of the earth. But if the salt loses its saltiness, how can it be made salty again? It is no longer good for anything, except to be thrown out and trampled by men. You are the light of the world. A city on a hill cannot be hidden. ... let your light shine before men, that they may see your good deeds and praise your Father in heaven.”

Chapter 6

The Adoption

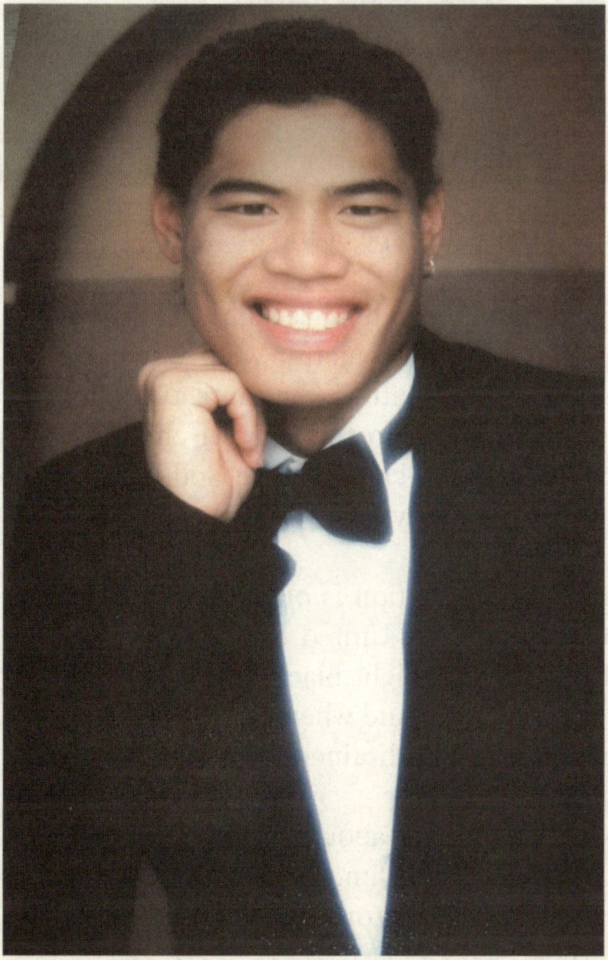

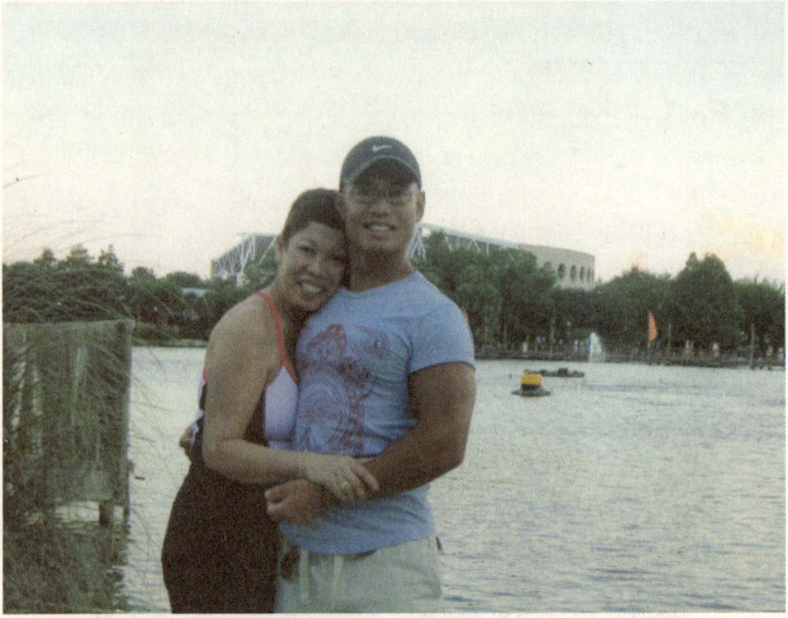

"With exemption for rape or incest ..."

That's what you most often hear in the abortion debate. It's the common ground no matter what your view or stance. Maybe instead of debating what an actual abortion is and what it actually does to the unborn child, we should all be on our hands and knees before God in prayer over this horrendous and divisive issue.

Abortion versus adoption is obviously an indelicate issue. Did you know in the United States, for every one white baby that's aborted, eight black babies are aborted? What should a woman do? And when it comes to rape—well, that is supposed to be a no-brainer.

What should we think about this as women, black, white, American Indian, Muslim, Jewish, Hindu, Puerto Rican, Korean, Asian, Catholic, or whatever other group you might belong to?

I am not the only person to carry the child of a rape to term. The child of the rapist did nothing wrong. As a Roman Catholic, I believe God imputes the soul when the egg is fertilized. A human being is now present. This much I know and believe. This is not above my pay grade. I am not asking anyone to follow me. I am not saying to vote for a Republican or a Democrat. Harry Reid, the senator from Nevada, is a Mormon and a Democrat and is strongly anti-abortion. This is not about knowing enough about politics. It's about knowing that a baby has a heartbeat and fingerprints after a few weeks.

Most people don't know what abortion is, how horrible it is, the silent scream of the baby. Once you know what it is, then you realize if you are human, you cannot go through with this abortion. Many have been tricked into it. Many have done this unknowingly. Others, of course, do this knowingly.

Regardless, if you are involved with abortion, you will suffer. Some say many addictions, like alcohol or drugs, can be traced to abortion. A country like South Korea, which has the lowest birth rate in the entire industrialized world and one of the highest rates of alcohol abuse, can stand as a testament to alcohol addiction and abortion.

I don't say this to make you feel bad. I say that if you left God out of the decision to have a baby and you chose an abortion, don't leave God out of the healing process that must take place. Moses murdered an Egyptian soldier. King David took Bathsheba sexually and then sent her husband off to die. Saul held Stephen's coat as he was stoned to death by rocks. Murderers have become great men of God. How many did Samson take down with him at the very end, even wearing chains, blinded, and doing the work of a donkey?

Most people know of Tim Tebow, the famous University of Florida quarterback who now plays in the NFL for the Denver Broncos. His mother had multiple abortions before he was born. I believe it was four or five. Imagine if Jesus Christ had been aborted. Imagine if Joseph had not been able to protect Baby Jesus and Mary on the run in Egypt while fleeing King Herod.

The previous is all the macro. What about the micro? How does a mother who is one of twelve siblings decide to give up her only precious son for adoption—this after raising and taking care of him for six years?

I guess I will have to back up a little bit and tell you about my time at the Subic Naval Base in the PI. You might have heard of this base, which was mentioned in the film *An Officer and a Gentleman*. There were contentious negotiations over the base between the United States and the Philippine government.

The Philippines, as you might know, were "discovered" by Magellan, who was killed there by Lapu-Lapu. Because of this, Magellan never circumnavigated the globe. The ship, which was named the *Victoria*, made it back to Europe without him. The Spanish colonized the PI, then the Americans, and then the Japanese. What, do we have a sign on our heads that says *"Come colonize us"?*

I colonized the garbage dump at Subic Bay. We stayed there for no more than two years. We were sheltered by an older couple, and there was hardly any food. The squalor and horrible living conditions made my son and me sick. There was no sanitation in place or running water. It is always either very hot or very muddy when it was monsoon season.

Eating expired canned goods was nauseating because we didn't know why they were thrown out. There were also some miscellaneous expired foods from the PX store. It is a place where they throw scrap metals that scavengers hunt to sell. Have you ever seen the movie *The Book of Eli?* It was kind of like that in a way, without all the that was portrayed in that moving film.

When my sister didn't come by to help us out because of extreme weather, we'd go hungry for days. Even my milk from my own body dried up. How do you explain that to your hungry baby? It was a case of trying to come home or die. I felt dead and neglected by God up in the mountains, so when my sister finally arrived, we decided to go back home with her to my older sister's place, which was in Manila.

But my sister's place was not the panacea I'd hoped for, nor the end of the rainbow. It was hard to make ends meet. Let's face it, this was the hardcore third world, and I was the poorest of the poor. I had to think about giving up my baby for adoption.

It was the hardest, most heart-wrenching decision I ever made, but it had to be done. Day and night I agonized over the decision for at least one year. How could I let go of my precious jewel? He was all I had, and he was my life.

Our financial situation has gotten worse. As noted, I just couldn't make ends meet, and he was always very sick. My plan to work as a housekeeper in the Middle East was also shut down. I failed my physical examination. They found a nodule in my thyroid, and I couldn't afford to have further testing to find out if it was malignant.

I was not employable in any place because I didn't have a college education. In the Philippines, you have to be college graduate to work even in a department store or food franchises. As a woman I was considered, since I was over the age of twenty-five, to be old.

I earned our daily living through buying and selling corn or other edible snacks. I would leave at 5:00 a.m. and go to the town, walk back, cook, and sell them around in the barrio. I would make profit equivalent of fifty cents. Woohoo! Most of the time that little bit of money was spent on food and medicine. I thought this is not the life I wanted for my son. I did not want him to suffer like I had. Please don't judge me too harshly. Even though I had been violently raped and left for dead, this baby represented the polar opposite of that. He represented all that was good in the world—at least to me.

Every night I'd go to the village chapel near our house. I would close the chapel's door, light a candle, and pray on my knees. I asked God to take my life if it would make my son's life better or to take both of our lives and end our hardship.

This was, of course, the coward's way out. Imagine asking God to take and kill in a rerun of Abraham and Isaac. How foolish I was. But I thought neither one of us deserved this miserable situation. My son was always teased around town for having no father, and the people looked down on me for having a son out of wedlock. Some kinder people did think I avoided shame and responsibility. I had been raped. How can people be so cruel? Who are they to judge, especially as Christians?

These are the people to whom Jesus will tell at the final

judgment, *"I never knew you ..."* The liars, frauds, users, those who take away and destroy what others build, those who go behind your back, those who are petty and jealous, untalented, and unwilling to admit any or all of these things, for that is a form of death to them. They go on with life, walking about as the living dead.

One day out of agony, I went to a church in the city and decided to go to confession. I thought perhaps this was what God wanted from me ... to confess to my sins. But what sins did I have? Smelling like a garbage dump? Eating expired foods from a can? Failing my physical? When I went to confession, I couldn't confess to anything. I just started crying my heart out. Little did I know that this was one of the turning points of my life. People attack the Catholic Church. They attack the Pope. They attack priests. But look at Indochina under Catholic rule versus the Khmer Rouge, the Pathet Lao, and the Vietcong.

There are positive elements to the Catholic Church—two thousand years worth of them.

The priest told me to come out of the box and instructed me to go the rectory and talk to him in person. He happened to be an American missionary. I told him my sufferings, from one thing to another since I was a child. I told him how heartbroken I was that my parents would not send me to school because we are poor. I told him about my many illnesses.

You already know this story of how I was diagnosed of leukemia when I was only fifteen years old. Then there was an infection of the liver because my parents couldn't afford the constant blood transfusions. I had to take herbal medication twenty-four hours a day. I was hospitalized in a government hospital with the interns playing *Dracula* and practicing on my veins to see who could draw blood the right way.

I told him the agony of being there in that hospital for three months with no visitors to come and see me. I told him about many patients dying around me every day. I told him about being raped and having my miraculous son out of that tragedy and how I was trying so hard to help us, even force us, to survive and just not making it.

I told him about many more difficulties and what I thought was God's punishment.

Anyway, after I poured out my soul to the priest, he said I could possibly be a saint and told me of the story of Job in the Bible. At that time, I didn't know who Job was. The priest told me that God won't punish good people, but like Job, I had been given many challenges. These challenges were not to punish me, but rather to share His cross and to see the "light." By this the priest meant that very special light that is of God and is always pointing the way to the narrow path toward the gates of heaven.

He also told me not to walk on my knees to the altar anymore. I could pray anywhere and I would be heard. He told me to learn to forgive in order to lighten the burden of my heart. He said that by doing so, this cognitive dissonance would help me focus on goodness of the Lord. Praying faithfully would also help me find the way out of my difficulties. The priest was showing his heart for the Lord—a heart of goodness—the reason why God had called him to this ministry. He was a soldier for God and for all good men and women, leading them to God and the cross through humility and goodness.

That moment I felt my spirit was lifted by many angels. This was the rallying point of my life and Christian faith. If you are reading this book as a Catholic, Protestant, Muslim, Jewish person, or even a Buddhist or nonbeliever, you will understand what I mean.

I went home lighthearted. I learned to finally forgive my brother, who had done so much that was cruel in my life by squandering my savings and introducing me to his friend who had evil intentions for my body.

Although our situation did not change, my attitude toward God changed. I found a personal relationship with God in my heart. I began to meditate prayerfully for all good things to come in His timetable. I completely relied on God for my strength to overcome my struggles and, when there were days when I couldn't go on, I just thought of how He was nailed on the cross for no fault of His own.

___ ___ ___

I was beginning to see the light at the end of my tunnel. Ideas came to my mind like, "Why not try find someone to adopt my son and so his life will change? Why not try to find another employer in the United States and try to go there to work?"

I ask my guardian angel for guidance, and I prayed to God about which way to go. My intuition was to do both, and I did just that.

I sent a letter to my former employers, who are both doctors in Pennsylvania, and asked them to tell my friend Carol of my hardship and situation with my son.

I was surprised to receive a letter from Carol detailing her sympathy and willingness to help me. She also offered to adopt my son and, should I agree, she promised that I would always be his mother and that I would never be denied the chance of knowing him as he grew up—if I ever made it back to the United States, that is.

I consulted with my brothers and sisters and also my parents. All of them discouraged me, especially my father. He said we would survive, just like all of us did. I was torn making the final decision. Yes, of course, we survived, but I looked at our miserable situation. I said to myself in a moment of reflection, *"This is not the life I want for my son. I want him to have security for his future and an education."*

I didn't have any security and, most of all my health was not so hot.

I made my final decision after praying day and night, always asking God to guide me which way to go. One evening after crying all night I wrote the go-ahead letter to Carol for her to make the arrangements to come to the PI so we could start the adoption proceedings.

My son's adoption story is very complex and even up to this very day, I am constantly hounded (or it is haunted?) by my decision. Was it the right thing to do under the pitiful circumstances? The decision broke my heart to pieces. Some say time heals a broken heart, but the scar of my child's adoption lingers on and, perhaps it always will until the end of my time on this planet.

I can tell you that it was the hardest paperwork I have ever had to obtain. I had to pay the local newspaper for an ad stating that my son was being given up for adoption.

Can you imagine what was going through my mind? I wonder what goes through the mind of a woman having an abortion, though, even after a rape.

This all happened during the monsoon season. I had to find the social worker assigned to my case, a woman who lived far away in some kind of no-man‘s land, and convince her that my son was an abandoned child and there was no means of support from anyone.

On top of it all, I had to convince her that her signature of approval was a matter of life and death for both me and my son. Most of all, I had to explain that her decision was our only hope of salvation. I guess the soaking rain over my body and my river of tears created compassion in her heart, because she signed the recommendation for adoption. (During this whole time, my son didn‘t know what was going on. He simply hugged me very tightly at night when we went to sleep).

I notified Carol of the approval, and in no time she came to the PI for the adoption proceedings. Convincing the judge was also extremely difficult, but my sad face and my tears always seem(ed) to work with God and human beings.

And so the process began, which would take another six months. When I say I was crying in this matter, I don‘t mean that I was an actress like Reece Witherspoon in A Far-Off Place. I just mean that I cried a lot and had a sad look on my face because I had been so broken most of the time. To have been raped and then raped again, left for dead, left for months on end in the hospital, living in the garbage dump at Subic Bay ... if you can't cry after all of that, then when can you cry?

What's the shortest verse in the Bible? "Jesus wept."

I had finally found God in the middle of my chaotic life. Miracles do happen when you least expect it. This miracle came in a form of a new employer to bring me back to United States—all expenses paid. All I had to do was to secure a visa from the United States Embassy. Securing a working visa is next to impossible, I was told. It would actually require a real miracle.

Luckily, my mother had a distant relative who worked in a travel agency in Manila and, with the money we borrowed to pay for the paperwork, I was given a tourist visa to enter the United States. I guess that's a little white lie that didn't hurt anyone, like *Forrest Gump's* mother told him.

— — —

As I noted, my son's adoption was a heart-wrenching, mind-boggling, and complex decision. When you have given your flesh and blood and you've been with your child for six years, day and night through hardship and illnesses, you would not only be broken by the decision of separation through adoption, but also so very afraid that it may not be the right decision for your child.

At a very young age, my son was a very sweet child. We had a mother-child bonding that ran deep. He did not want to see me crying and always hugged me ever so tightly when he saw that I was in tears. He always thought I was in pain because I always said I had a stomachache. Of course, it was never physical pain, but the pain of uncertainty, our future, his future. If you want pain, then try multiple rapes and leukemia. So, dear reader, you might be asking what happened to my son.

Before I can go on with my son's story, where he was conceived, where he was born, and his first two years, I feel that you should know the whole connection of how I found his adoptive single parent. Without this chronicle of events, this book will leave you with unanswered questions.

Let's go back to the time to when I came home from the United States after staying five years with my first employers, who were both doctors in Chambersburg, Pennsylvania.

When I thought I had saved enough money to start a small business in the Philippines, I ask my oldest brother to start a business for me. I sent him all my savings, and he started a bakeshop in Metro Manila, where he lived at that time. I was very confident that it was successful, as I received letters from my sisters that my brother became rich overnight. I also was told that he opened another business, a beer garden. A beer garden is a karaoke bar that has women working as "hospitality girls." They can sit down with men if requested and make commission on the beer they serve.

I was so eager to come home to start a new beginning. My stay with the doctors and their three daughters made me very homesick and depressed for five years, as I was not able to have a social life. The only friendship I developed during that time period was with Carol, one of my employers' friends. She was a nurse who was also employed at the same hospital where the doctors worked.

Carol is much older than me, but we got along fine. She picked me up once a week to clean her apartment, and then we would play scrabble. After that, we either went to dinner or a movie. We became close friends and, when I left, she even gave me going-away gift and some money. I thought she was very kind and generous.

I did not yield to the doctors‘ wishes that I stay with them. Five years was very hard on me emotionally, and the thought of staying longer for the sake of their children caused me to have many sleepless nights. I missed my parents, my siblings, and my home.

At that time in the mid-1970s, people were just talking about the "information superhighway." There were no immediate forms of communication except cablegram and telephone. Since my parents lived in the province, my only way of letting them know about my trip home was the cablegram. The doctors sent it for me.

I flew from JFK Airport and, after flying twenty hours with two four-hour stopovers, I arrived at the former Manila International Airport. It was a very long, strenuous flight, and I looked forward to seeing throngs of relatives pick me up. I waited and waited for what like seemed forever.

After two hours of waiting and there was no one to pick me up, I panicked and started crying. *How could they not show up?* I was not only exhausted, but I was also very scared. I didn‘t know my way around in Manila, and I didn‘t know how to get to my brother‘s or my sister‘s house.

A Good Samaritan, a taxi driver, noticed my situation and approached me. He said he was short of one more passenger in his cab and asked if I would like to share a ride. I didn't have any choice but to accept his offer. I told him that I only knew the address of the closest place I could go, my sister's house in Pasay City. He told me my sister's address was on the way to his other passenger's destination and to not worry about being kidnapped or held up by thieves and robbers in the area, as he would make sure I arrived safely to where I was going.

I arrived at my sister's house, and it was probably combination of joy and feeling sorry for me that made all of them cry. My younger brother Dodo and my younger sister Cecilia were there, and we all kissed and hugged. They hadn't received the cablegram. It arrived one week later.

I rested for a day and immediately asked my older sister to help me find my oldest brother to find out the status of the business he started for me.

The sad story began as we were on the bus on the way to my brother. My sister Lolita said, "I don't think you have any money left. Arnold started a beer garden and restaurant, and he lost a lot of money gambling and womanizing at the same time." I said, "It cannot happen. The money I sent was for my future, so it was my blood, my sweat, and my tears. No way!" No dream of mine would go down the drain.

I was hopeful when I finally met up with Arnold. Then I heard the truth ... there was very little money left and it was tied up in the beer garden business. I told him to sell it even at a loss so I could start a new beginning.

The business was sold, and from the proceeds, I started a small bakeshop. It was very hard, as I had to get up 4:00

a.m. to open the shop and then stay late to continue selling until there were no more customers. This operation was open seven days a week, and it was only me and my baker running it. Although I was working very hard and putting in long hours, I was not making any profit.

Arnold told me he suspected I was being robbed by my baker at night or at dawn just before I come to the store. When I questioned my baker about missing supplies, he immediately resigned and went away.

I had to close the bakeshop while my brother looked for the baker‘s replacement. It was not a pretty picture. I was doomed to fail. I was running out of money and, most of all, I was running out of hope. I did not anticipate the ongoing bad situation in my life.

One day my brother introduced me to one of his friends. His name was Rick, and I was told he was a good baker. He said he could help me restart the bakeshop and he would do most of the work . He would not only make all the bread and cakes, but he would also stay and sell them so I could have my break in the afternoon. I was working fourteen to sixteen hours day, and it was taking a toll on me. I was always so exhausted and began to hate what I was trapped into doing. Rick was a big help, and he became my friend.

One day he said, “You should have a day off. Close the bakeshop mid-afternoon and I will take you sightseeing near the US Subic Naval Base in Zambales province.” I agreed because I thought he was trustworthy and we were going as friends.

It was to be the beginning of more misfortunes. I was so naive and did not ask questions. My first mistake was not knowing the location and how far it would take us to get there by bus. The second mistake was not knowing there was curfew in Manila past 10:00 p.m. We left after 2:00 p.m. It took more than five hours to get there. Because we were passing beautiful scenery, peaks and valleys, I did not pay attention to the time.

When we arrived at our destination, it was already getting dark. There was really nothing else to see but strip clubs where most American marines and officers hung out at night. I saw many Americans walking around with Filipina women as their escorts. I was not comfortable in the environment, so I asked Rick to take me back home. I told him I was very disappointed with the trip and I didn‘t like the club atmosphere of the town.

He became angry and said there was no way we could go back that night, as there was no more transportation running to Manila at that time. Even if there was, we ran the possibility of getting arrested under the current Marcos Martial Law declaration.

My heart sunk to the ground. Again I had that feeling that I was doomed and something terrible was about to happen, and it did. Rick convinced me to check into a cheap motel for the night, and he promised that we could leave first hour the buses were allowed to go back to Manila. I agreed because I did not have any choice.

The unthinkable happened as he walked me to my room. He did not leave, and he forced himself on me. He was a monster disguised as a lamb. I screamed and fought back very hard, but nobody came to my rescue. It seemed that screaming and fighting were a regular occurrences in that horrendous place—but those women were getting paid. I was there being violated. This horrible and despicable motel is a "house of sin," and I was there against my will. I will not elaborate on the cruelty I suffered, as it pains me to recall the event. All I knew that moment was that I was again neglected by God and my angels. If they were there, they would not have allowed the devil to destroy me. I wished I had died that night. I lost all my reasons to live. It was the longest night of agony I ever endured, worse than my nights at Philippine General Hospital in Manila when at age of fifteen years I was confined for months and surrounded with dying patients every day and had no visitors.

Over and over I wished and prayed that I die that moment. Again, God did not listen to me, and I lived to tell you my story. I must be the chosen one to share the lesson of brokenness, patience, and perseverance.

The rape was all planned. Rick even had a hideout where I virtually was prisoner for two months. He was not working and eventually became short of money, so he forced me to pawn all the jewelry I had been wearing. I learned later on that he found buyers and sold each piece of my valuable jewelry and later on also sold my favorite camera.

To make matter worse , the despicable acts committed against me day after day made me miss my monthly period, and I began to have horrible morning sickness. When Rick discovered I could be pregnant, he beat me up so severely hoping I would have a miscarriage. It did not happen, for which I am so thankful. As a Catholic, I am against abortion.

I badly needed help and, when he left to buy some food, I escaped. I found a couple living not to too far away from my imprisonment. I told them my story and they decided to help me find a place where I could stay temporarily. They took me to another couple who lived near the garbage dump at the US Subic Naval Base. Their means of livelihood was scavenging scrap metals and waste refuse from the navy military and residents of the base.

You might ask why I did not go to the proper authorities to report the rape and the abused. I did go to the police, but I was not taken seriously. It was a "date rape," and I have no witnesses, so there was no case. There was nothing like that in their book. It was a waste of their time.

What I did find was not a shock to me. Rick had a long record of battery and assault, among other things, like theft. The police also told me that even if I had a solid case, they could not arrest him because they don't have any more room at the city jail.

At that time I was told they arrested activists instead, people who rallied against Marcos and his cronies. Those who were against Marcos got jail time, not criminals like Rick. The whole Philippine justice system was upside down. You know it by the imprisonment of the former Senator Benigno Aquino. His only crime was that he loved the people and his country and he suffered too much and even lost his life at the end.

I was resigned to my pitiful fate and scraped some money to be able to see my younger sister Cecilia, who worked as a waitress in Manila. I asked for financial help because I could not go home to my parents' house. She told me that all of them were worried and looked for me when I was missing for months. I told her where she could come and visit me while I was waiting for my baby to be born. When I described the place, she said, "Oh my Lord! The jeep we hired to look for you broke down exactly above you." They could have found me, but I guess God has other plans for me to make me suffer more. That was my belief then, as everything in my life changed for the better.

My sister continued to make the trip to visit me until I gave birth to my son. I was also told that when she learned I was pregnant, my mother did not care to see me anymore. So problems upon problems were piled on top of me. Crying buckets of tears was my everyday life day after day.

Because my son and I had poor nutrition, we both became ill. My son became asthmatic, and my anemic condition came back. When my sister came, I said good-bye to the nice couple, thanked them profusely for sheltering us, and prayed that they too would be able to leave that no-man's land.

My son and I stayed with my older sister in Pasay City, and I tried to find a job, but I was not employable. My sister Lolita had three very young children at that time, and it was difficult to make ends meet, let alone for my son and me to add to their tight budget. The only solution was to come home to my parents and ask for their forgiveness.

That was the only solution I could see in our bleak horizon. After spending few months at my sister Lolita's house, we came home.

My mother did not welcome me with open arms, but she

immediately fell in love with my son, who was about two years old at the time. Being at my parents' house was more comfortable than anywhere else, and I made a pledge to myself and my son that we would not be hungry again. Because I really worked hard, we managed to buy food on a regular basis, allowing us to eat on time.

It was extremely hard to understand what was going on in our lives. My son continued to be sickly, and every penny I saved was spent on his medicine. I could not imagine how we could go on with our hand-to-mouth situation. I often thought and prayed for a better way of living.

For many years I was torn by my decision of giving him up for a better life. I cried silently at night and wished for him to look for me, as I didn't know where he was.

My wish came true after fourteen years. Armand, as I named him, sent me a letter and his pictures. My heart jumped with joy. Tears of happiness rolled down my cheeks.

My husband and I hugged each other, and we both thanked God for His blessing.

In the letter he requested to see me. He said he would like to come to New Jersey and stay if I wished. He also said he could come right away if I sent him an airplane ticket. He gave me his address and a phone number to call.

When I called Armand, no words came out of my mouth. I was speechless and could not remember all the beautiful words I wanted to say in his growing-up years. I could not express all the mother's love I had in my heart—the love that was never given because I was denied motherhood.

All I was able to say was, "I missed you so much, and it will be a joy to have you back in my life." I also told him to give me his other name and his address so I could send him the plane ticket.

My husband booked and paid for Armand's ticket. He was coming from Fort Myers, Florida, and arriving at the Newark Airport at 6:00 p.m. The date was December 15, and it was also the last day for me to accomplish my Pacesetter goal. I need to sell $3,000 in one day to secure my status as one of the top sellers in our store. I would normally work long hours during holiday season, but that particular day was so special because I hadn't seen and hugged my precious baby for such a long time.

I was on the edge the day before my son's arrival. I was nervous about him arriving on the same day I was trying very hard to make my goal. Every sale and every moment counted. I was being pulled in two directions. All I needed was one probe of, "Yes, I can become Pacesetter seven years in a row before 5:00 p.m. and run to the airport to meet my precious child."

I made my goal just before 5:00. Thank God the store manager made the announcement before the store opened. He said I was trying to make my goal on that eventful day and if employees and managers needed to shop, to shop with me. Most people in the store who knew about my son's surfacing out of the blue came to my rescue and did their Christmas shopping. I believe in God, and I believe my prayers were answered that day.

Luke 1:37 says, "For nothing is impossible with God."

My husband picked me up, and we rushed to the airport. We hardly talked on the way. He held my hand every so often and just keep saying, "Everything is going to be all right." He knew I was afraid of how things were going to be with me and my son.

It was a joyful event for me when I finally saw him. He was still cute in my eyes, but as a grown young man, he was incredibly handsome. I cried. He hugged and embraced me, and off we went out to eat. There was so much to catch up on, but there was a nagging feeling inside me that something was not right. My husband did most of the talking, as Armand and I became so tongue-tied to speak to each other. There was a tear in my heart that I could not discern.

My fear later on manifested in our mother-son relationship. My blood that circulated through his body had no more significance. He had no family feelings for me. It broke my heart when he openly said he could not call me Mom, because he already had one. He came because he was curious about who I was and he wanted to know why he and Carol had to leave the first home he learned to love. He came to tell me how hurt he was that he had to leave his friends because I was harassing Carol at her place of employment. He also said his grandmother lost a lot of money because they had to sell their house immediately at a low cost so they could get away from me. It was doubly painful to be told by my own son that I did something wrong when, all along, it was the other way around. Carol lied and completely took him away from me.

I cared so much about him, and I continued to be understanding of his ways. Carol spoiled him rotten. At nineteen years of age, Armand didn't know how to do laundry and how to cook or do simple things like vacuum and clean his room.

The worst thing I discovered was very disappointing. At a very young age, his credit was already ruined. I found out when I tried to help him open a checking account, the bank denied his application. I was torn to pieces because I believe having a good credit is also a part of financial success.

My husband took his time to talk to him and tried to explain to him all the sacrifices I made to get him come to the United States. He also told Armand about the praying and all the waiting I did for the day he would come back to my life. I know Lou tried many times to show him we really cared, but things just did not work out.

The straw that broke the camel‘s back happened when I gave him my credit card. He immediately spent more than $ 3,000 in less than one hour. He bought miscellaneous components for his car and also a gym membership for a girl he had just met. I learned about it when I told my friend I had given my son a credit card just before I came to work. She told me that was a big mistake and I should cancel the card right away. When I called the bank, there were charges already incurred, and I hated myself for not being a part of a solution. I became a contributor to my son‘s problem.

I made a painful decision to let him go again. This time my decision is based on "tough love." I told him that, although I loved and cared for him so much, he had to go back to Carol because I could not tolerate irresponsibility and flagrant disobedience. I also said my home would always be open for him whenever he decided to change his ways.

When he left, he left me with a broken heart. All my dreams for him became suspended in the dark clouds of doubt and despair. I asked myself again if it might have been better to just left him in the Philippines to grow up surrounded by my kin and in a more conservative environment.

My husband said I made the best decision at the time and that I should not have any regrets, as I made a supreme sacrifice and the most unselfish decision a mother could for the sake of her child.

I love him so much, but there is really nothing I can do to fix his life's various problems. There are no perfect people or sons, for that matter. I want him to learn on his own. I tried very hard to correct my friend's mistake of spoiling him so much, but there's a saying that goes, "You can only bend a tree while it is still young." He was spoiled to a point of destruction and, until he finds his way out, I am helpless. I cannot undo the damage that has been done. I have to live with this. I can pray. That much I can do ...

He is very appreciative of what I did to get him to where he is now in life and always says so. But I believe that love is active. I have to be tough with him when I see him, although it kills me as a mom. I only want the best for his future. He can own my resort at anytime, but I'd rather turn it into a foundation to aid poor and sick people, as I know giving the resort to him will only do more harm.

He is still in Fort Myers, Florida, and I meet with him occasionally.

I want him to become a man worthy of my own hopes, goals, and dreams. I want him to be a man of drive, courage, kindness, and goodness. I want him to be man after God's own heart like King David. I pray for this every day. It is important that parents live moral lives for their young and impressionable children and grandchildren. I know I am not a perfect person. I don't claim to have all the answers. But I know prayer is a great answer.

Chapter 7

The Grace of giving (My sister Cecilia's Story)

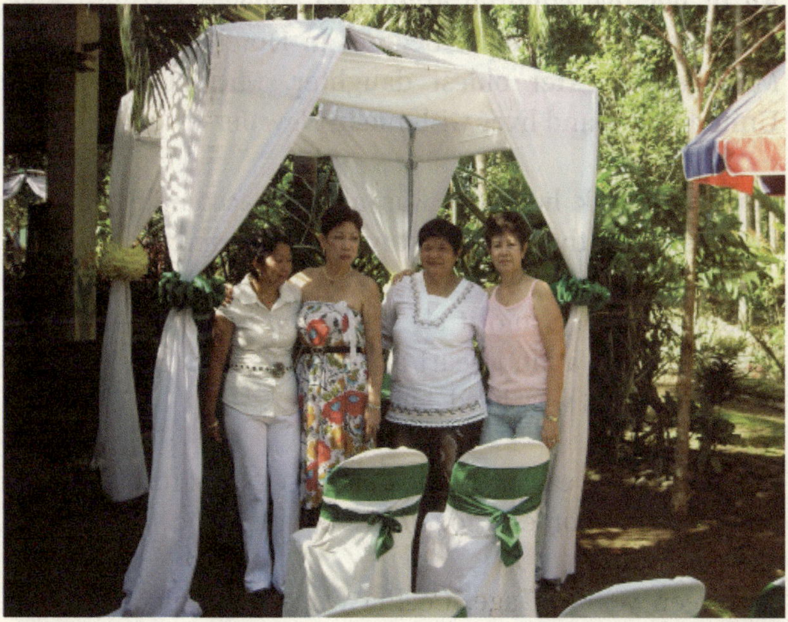

Always risk in faith because God multiplies. The lesson can be found in 2 Corinthians 9:10: "Now he who supplies seed to the sower and bread for food will also supply and increase your store of seed and will enlarge the harvest of your righteousness."

God asks for faith. He wants us to sacrifice in advance, not knowing what we will get in return.

My sister, Cecilia, did what God commands us to do. She helped and gave to me till it hurt, and now she is receiving the grace of giving.

Cecilia, like me, is well on her way to becoming a millionaire. She lives in a mansion worth five million pesos and has a thriving catering business, equipment, and automobiles that are worth beyond her wildest dreams.

All of her five children graduated college. Two are RNs, and three have bachelor degrees in Hotel and Restaurant Management. Her oldest daughter, Michelle, is in the United States and lives with me in New Jersey.

You might ask how she was able to accomplish all her dreams, when the family history is of extreme poverty.

This is her story, and it all started with her generosity of spirit. She has a kind heart and a brave soul. She dared to dream, worked very hard, and did it.

As I mentioned earlier, all my siblings, except for Susan, the youngest, left home to go to different places to work.

At fifteen years of age, Cecilia went to Manila and lived with my older sister Lolita. She did light housekeeping and babysitting for my nieces and nephews while she studied high school. After she graduated high school, she found a job at one of the international chain restaurants in Quezon City, one hour away from Manila. She was making good money in wages in tips and was able to live on her own.

During this time, many unfortunate cruel events were happening in my life, and we didn't have a way of communicating with each other. The distance between us was very far, six hours each way.

Driven by her dream and ambition to finish college, she went to night school to pursue a business education.

That dream was cut short because I needed desperate help. I was six months pregnant from the rape, and the couple, who was helping me, needed financial help themselves. Rummaging through the Dumpster for food and scrap metals was not sustaining all our miserable existence. We were short of food most of the time.

I borrowed money and took the bus. I went to my sister Lolita first, but at that time, she was also going through financial crisis. There was no way she could afford to help me, so I turned to Cecilia instead.

I told her my predicament and where she could find me, living with a couple of scavengers up in the mountains near the former Subic Naval Base.

After we hugged and cried, I left with a heavy heart and a high hope that she would come to my rescue.

At that time my parents completely gave up on looking for me. I'd rather live in miserable conditions than let them see me in that sorry state of my life.

Cecilia came and fulfilled her promise. She came devotedly in all types of weather, heavy storms, thunder and lightning. She came bringing me money, groceries and, later on, baby clothes.

Our added expenses put a strain on Cecilia's college education. She could not afford both, so she gave up school and chose me.

This went on for months that turned into almost two years. What a noble sacrifice my sister was making for me. I promised myself that, God willing and my life turned around, I would repay all her goodness and more.

I finally had my son, and things got worse for us. We were both in poor health because of poor nutrition and lack of food. I did not have a choice but to ask my sister Lolita if we could stay in their house in Manila temporarily.

Our life was not great there either. We were living in a cramped dwelling, and it was extremely hot and uncomfortable in Manila during the summer season, flooded all over during the rainy season.

In the meantime, Cecilia fell in love, got married, and started a family. I heard bad news about her husband. I'm quite sure he did not start that way, because I know my sister is too smart to fall for the wrong person. I was told that her husband is a drug addict, a womanizer, and a wife beater. All that bad news broke my heart to pieces.

The good news came when I was told that my mother had forgiven me for having a son out of wedlock. Everyone thought it was my fault, and people looked at me just as the people in the Bible looked at Mary Magdalene.

I just looked at our situation on a day-to-day basis and

considered my suffering a chance to share the life of Jesus, who was crucified on the cross and died for the sake of mankind.

If there was a divine reason for what I went through, it was truly obscured and there was no visible sign of relief in sight for me to be hopeful. Even then, I continued to pray and believe God would deliver me from all the evil happening to me and around me.

I'm anchored in my faith, and my belief system is embedded in my heart and my soul. From reading the Bible, I learned it contains the complaints of other human beings before us who became discouraged over the unfairness of this life. God did not promise them that He would make their life better immediately.

Job and Jeremiah were both biblical complainers. Both of their lives got worse before they became better, and it is the same with my life.

God did not promise us a life of health, wealth, and happiness, free from suffering and discomfort. I knew in my heart that one day soon this too would come to pass, and it did.

Going back to Cecilia's story, I must say she reaped what she sowed. Her seeds of goodness multiplied. Although I can never measure the amount she has given me, I repaid her back in amounts immeasurable to anyone's standard and will continue to do for so long as I shall live.

How did I do it? I prayed and kept a positive attitude despite my difficult situation, and it finally paid off.

Things of God started to fall on my life, one after the other. First, I found an employer to bring me back to the United States to work as their babysitter-housekeeper in New Jersey. Second, my employer informed me that my friend Carol wanted to help me by adopting my son, promising that should I make it to the United States, I would not be denied my motherhood; I would always be my son's mother.

I was able to come to the United States immediately, leaving my son at my sister Lolita's house, as his adoption papers and visa were being processed, which would take another six months.

I was allowed by my new employers to pick up additional jobs as long as I was able to keep up with my responsibilities of housekeeping. I was able to work at a deli for few hours a day and babysit the daughters of the next-door neighbors overnight. The parents worked the graveyard shift, and they came home just around 7:00 a.m., which was perfect timing for me to start my housekeeping chores at my employer's house next door.

I saved all my earnings and was able to offer Cecilia relief from her bad marriage. I knew in my heart that if I didn't do anything to save and help her, her children would not have a chance for a better future.

I told her to leave her husband immediately and come home and live with my parents. She did and there, at the barrio, I gave her financial support and subsidized a small grocery store for her not to be totally dependent on me. This continued on for many years till her oldest daughter, Michelle, graduated from high school. Immediately after graduation, I planned to help her come to the United States.

My plan materialized when my other niece, Mary Jean, aided me in getting her a diplomatic visa from a Middle Eastern Ambassador who worked for the United Nation at the time.

Mary Jean is the third daughter of my sister Lolita. She was recruited to work as an administrative assistant to an UAE Ambassador in New York, and her connection opened up all kinds of possibilities for the future of all her cousins, Cecilia's five children.

Oh, the tangled web I created for the glory of God. I have to be creative and resourceful in all my decisions concerning the future of all my loved ones.

I made a promise that none of my remaining siblings would have to go through what I've been through and I would deliver them from the hardships of poverty and ignorance.

Michelle finished her contract with the ambassador, and then she lived with me. I taught her everything I know and encouraged her to dare to dream and do it with all her might. I gave her my wisdom and life's philosophies to get ahead in life. I told her that she had two choices. First, she could enjoy first and suffer later, or second, she could suffer first and enjoy later.

I told her that I chose to suffer first and she could witness the fruit of my labor and sacrifices. I am well ahead in life, and the lessons to be learned are in front of her eyes, from "shoeless and no suitcase Julie" to owner of a beautiful resort and many other prized real estate properties here in the United States and in the Philippines.

My niece took my advice. She also worked two or three jobs at a time and saved half of her earnings. She sent half of the money she made to my sister and, because of Michelle's effort, all her siblings were able to finish high school and then college, one after the other. At the same time, Cecilia was very courageous and started a catering business, which grew rapidly in no time. She slowly built an empire from a humble twenty-piece chair rental to a huge multi-catering company.

She and I shared the same resolved love and commitment to our family, and that made both of us winners, not only in the eyes of many people, but also in the eyes of God.

We both risked in faith, and God multiplied our blessings.

Chapter 7

Sand(y) through the Hourglass

I believe in angels. I know and feel in my heart that they are sent to us by God to assist us here on Earth for various reasons.

All my life I'd been looking for angels, and I found some that really made difference in my existence on this blue and green orb floating in space.

The angels I met helped me change the course of my life. I found out that some angels come in human form (the missionary priest, my husband, my journalist/professor friend LoBaido) or they come to me in spirit, helping me to decide which way to go.

If there was ever a time when I needed an angel, it was when my niece Sandy was still alive. She died of an undiagnosed blood disorder only a few days before her eighteenth birthday. She was the oldest child of my youngest sister, Susan.

From the time of Sandy's birth, she had been hospitalized a few times each year for bleeding. Sometimes her bleeding was external and the solution was much simpler, as my sister and her husband would always find donors to donate blood for transfusions. Other times the bleeding was more difficult to treat. This was when she would bleed internally, mostly near her joints. This was always very painful because she would have to undergo surgery and be confined to the hospital.

Sandy suffered so much pain from the time she was a baby. The pediatrician found her bleeding early on her umbilical cord. It took an abnormal amount of time to heal. The onset of her health problems came right there and then.

Of course, the monetary burden of her illness took a toll on my sister and brother in terms of finances. Up to this day, the family is struggling financially and I am always there to help them out—be it with money, food, and/or medicine.

They literally became homeless until I gave them the beautiful house I built for my parents. I gave it to them just after my parents died, which was not that long ago.

Sandy's illness was a mystery to all the doctors who had the opportunity to try to cure her. They could not find any diagnosis from all the extensive blood and laboratory work. All they could do was shake their heads in exasperation.

Sandy was a beautiful child with an angelic face, kind and sweet. One could not help but fall in love with her. Like me, she was always in the top of her class although she missed one-third of her school years due to her illness. Like me, she also dreamed of finishing school and eventually pursuing a college education. It was a dream that was harder and harder to realize as her internal bleeding occurred more and more often and her health struggles intensified.

All the bad news broke my heart and pained me so much. It was not the pain from helping my sister financially, but feeling Sandy's pain—the surgeries, the blood transfusions, and the loneliness of being in the hospital. If you recall from what you've read earlier in this book, I, myself, had been in the same predicament many years before, so I know what it is like. However, I had no visitors to come and see me in the hospital for months on end. This you also know. All of this should drive us ever closer to Jesus.

I prayed for a miracle, and I waited. I also prayed for her angels to offer up some kind of human, physical, and even miraculous intervention. My hope was that there's an angel out there somewhere just waiting to be found. I speak of an angel in human form that a celestial angel might in turn find and bring into the lives of myself and my niece Sandy.

I did research via the Internet for her illness and contacted various laboratories who apparently claimed they did or could do clinical trials on new drugs for unknown blood disorders. Most of the time none offered help. Sometimes they just couldn't offer an answer. Sandy's problem seemed beyond space age medical science. You might recall the story in the New Testament of Jesus healing someone who had a blood disorder. To be sure, such disorders have been around for thousands of years. In the Middle Ages they were still bleeding people with leeches.

I was so desperate. I became very aggressive about asking for help. Sometimes through our prayers we have to create our own miracles.

On one particularly faith-filled morning, I decided to e-mail my journalist/professor friend in Korea. I did not know him personally, as we had only corresponded through the Internet. He was a world-renowned journalist and, at that time, was also a professor teaching journalism, mass communication, and advanced globalization studies courses, in addition to conducting training with top-level South Korean military officers.

I had put an ad on the Internet for a future ESL school at my resort in the Philippines, and he responded. His résumé was amazingly impressive. I was in awe of his amazing accomplishments and, I must admit, of the famous and important people he knows.

I thought, in my desperation, I would take a wild shot in the dark in a quest to find a medical connection through him. I thought he would know all the best people in the world, since he had been in forty-two countries and had published a book on the Kurds and more than 338 factual and intellectual articles at WND.com. I was hoping he would know a doctor or that he might know someone (anyone) who could ,in turn, connect me with the right person who could help Sandy.

Much to my surprise, it was noble of him to put me in contact with his doctor friend in Ojai, California (a fine, brilliant devout, Catholic doctor schooled at the elite Washington University in St. Louis, Missouri), who put me in contact with a blood specialist in Oregon.

I started corresponding through e-mail with both doctors. I supplied both of them with Sandy's complete blood reports from her previous hospitalizations. Since the doctor from Oregon found that the blood report was inconclusive, I was told that the solution was to bring Sandy to United States. I told them that Sandy needed sponsorship papers to obtain a medical visa to come. Otherwise she would not be allowed.

My request was construed as asking for charity and handouts, like people on welfare here in the United States, so a kind of painful refusal went back and forth through the digital world of e-mail. It was a total insult to my pride, as I have never been on public assistance. As I explained earlier in this book, I have always saved enough money by working two or even three jobs to secure my future.

I stopped corresponding with this doctor's office manager immediately. Luckily, due to my further research, I found a blood disorder organization in the United States, and they were very helpful in every aspect of my request for more information. I will never forget their kindness, even to a total stranger. There are still so many good people in the world who strive for heroism every day. This is why God is so longsuffering with mankind. There are angels celestial and angels human/terrestrial. Of this I have no doubt.

The doctor, who is the director of the blood disorder organization was very helpful and put me in contact with a blood specialist in Manila, who incidentally, was Sandy's hematologist at the University of Saint Thomas Hospital. I placed an overseas phone call to her and organized the details of an impending appointment for Sandy when I got home.

I kept my journalist/professor friend informed of what was going on. In the meantime, he was also trying hard on his end.

My admiration toward my friend grew each day because of his unconditional effort and kindness. Since he is single, I prayed then and still pray that he will find the woman of his dreams who can make his heart smile.

I planned my vacation just to be able to take care of Sandy's illness once and for all, meaning I didn't care how much it would cost or what it would take.

Our appointment with her doctor was for a Saturday. She passed away the Wednesday just before that Saturday. Just when her life was almost in my grasp, she left and went to heaven. Sandy's sudden death broke me to pieces, and I cried loudly without shame.

I took care of her cold body and put her makeup on. I thought I saw her smile at me as I took her picture. Yes, although she had been in pain, there was a smile in her face. Her suffering was gone. The uncertainty of her life was gone. Her eternity had begun.

I took her death as an indication that she had been saved from all the other complications of financial burdens and also to save her parents and siblings further hardship in all aspect of her illness.

Chapter 9

God Is the Light I Follow

When people see me with a huge smile on my face most of the time, they think my life is perpetually happy.

Yes, my life is now amazing, but it is far from perfect. God is not finished with me yet. He is still brewing me to perfection.

Yes, I went through extreme illnesses, leukemia, infection of the liver, and hemorrhagic fever and survived. I am still fighting another battle, and it is a constant struggle to remain a winner.

Ten years ago, I had a major gynecological female surgery, and the result was catastrophic to my hormonal glands. I had a chemical imbalance that impaired reasoning capabilities in my brain. It happened so quickly I didn‘t realized what hit me till I couldn‘t function anymore.

To explain it bluntly, I completely lost my mind. I found myself crying for no reason and snapping at very slight provocation from customers at work.

I was not getting along with my coworkers and always felt everyone was working against me. It was always a struggle for me to even get up in the morning and go to work. Nothing mattered anymore. I was always very depressed and mad at myself for feeling so grossly miserable every day.

My poor husband suffered with me, and we both decided I needed help. My primary care physician recommended that I go for counseling and prescribed medication for me.

The medication did not help, and I went into downward spiral emotionally.

To protect my job and my reputation as a vested customer service all star, I voluntarily quit my job and tried all kinds of anti-depression pills to find a cure.

It was the hardest time of my life as I was trying to survive my illness. Why bad things happen to good people like me was always a never-ending question to God.

Another bad thing that happened was the wrong medication given to me. The side effect caused me to have suicidal tendencies, and I cried in pain of for life.

One day, I was alone, and my thinking was clouded heavily by the drug. I called my doctor and said I didn‘t want to live anymore. Honestly, I didn‘t want to die, but I was too scared and too tired to live.

My doctor called 911, and the police came immediately. They also called my husband at work, and he followed the ambulance the police sent for me. I was guarded for twenty-four hours until I was out of the critical period.

It was a defining moment for me. How did I lose myself?

Why did God leave me on my own? How did I lose the Light I follow? Was this another endurance test?

The doctors explained that our brains are as much a part of our body as any part that gets sick or damaged. Both the neurologist and the psychiatrist said I could pray all I wanted but I needed to be given the right medication to have my brain heal and function properly.

I listened to their advice and took my medication religiously. I also went on a four-year sabbatical from working at my department store.

I went back to the Philippines and spent my time developing the property I bought for my husband and my retirement.

There I found the passion of my heart. I gardened from the first burst of sunlight to dusk, and at night, I watched the birds fly in the pale moonlight. I found my heaven on earth, and most of all, I found my true self. I am not dead; I am so alive!

I found my peace and my inner strength again. I found the Light I follow. I found the reason why these things happen. He wanted me to see what I was living for and my divine reason of existence.

I needed to share my blessings with those unfortunate people around me. He broke me to see the needs of other less fortunate. He wanted me to see that there are other colors in the rainbow, and things of God are found in the road less traveled.

I needed to go back to the Philippines to share my gift of

nature. I needed to invite the homeless children of Manila and have them camp at my resort every year. I needed to have the Youth for Christ Ministry camp and spread the gospel of the Lord. I needed to show people how one person can make a difference one person at a time.

I thank God for my bipolar illness. It brought me closer to God again.

Final Thoughts

For you, my dear reader, and to God Almighty, I want to thank you for taking the time to buy and read this book. I want to donate all the income from this book to help the indigent people in my barrio and also to have scholarships for children of parents who cannot afford to send them to school. I wanted, but I needed to continue the free yearly medical mission at my resort.

I ask nothing for myself. That's also my philosophy in life—to give your all, always, and leave it to God to see when and how you are paid back.

In this book I detailed for you my late father's problems. He was a carpenter and tried to build things, but he also tore them down with gambling. Yet, that could not take away his genius. He was a sinner like the rest of us. If he is an angel looking down on me, that would be a great thing.

The Bible says, "There is more joy in heaven for one sinner repented than a thousand righteous."

Don't pity me for my two years in a garbage dump. Ask yourself if you live in one right now. You might live in the Taj Mahal, but could still be sitting in a garbage dump in various other ways. We all fall short of the glory of God, and God is no respecter of persons.

I was raped not once, but twice and left for dead. I was violated, but how many violate all tenets of moral purity, live in multi-generational sexual immorality, and shamelessly parade this in front of their own children and grandchildren without conscience? If you feel this is wrong, then this is a good thing. It means there is a little voice inside telling you it is wrong. Change your life. Make your stand like the characters in the novel, *The Stand*. Forgive yourself as you forgive others. Just know that God rejoices in any movement toward righteous living. If you seek sanctification, you will feel God's power.

I had leukemia and was abandoned and left alone in the hospital, but God raised me up. I wanted to die, but God showed me the way to life came by passing through, not around, the trials the Lord Himself faced on Earth. I worked for little money, but now I am halfway to being a millionaire. It is once again the case of the turtle versus the rabbit.

Piece by piece I bought the land for my resort. I got back all the land my father had lost by gambling. I worked so hard. My planning, my sweat, my risk, and my ingenuity continued along without hesitation.

I want you all to do the same. I want you to believe in yourself, make a plan, and then take tiny and concrete steps toward your goals.

One day not long ago it was so beautiful outside—sunny and bright and seemingly not like winter at all. I was looking outside the window while ironing what I would wear that day, a beautiful flowered dress. I thought of these words: "Bloom where you are planted."

This is one of my favorite quotations. (Of course, we should be looking to create our own quotations and experience God directly and not through other people.) It tells me that wherever you are in your stage in life, you should love what you are doing and grow in the direction of your dreams. Follow the sun, follow your intuition, and listen for quiet direction in your heart of hearts.

Do not be afraid to take risks. Prayers can cement your belief, so be patient and wait. Eventually you will reap the flowers of your perseverance. The garden that God would seek to plant in my heart blooms every day. I have a beautiful life, just like the rose garden.

God pruned my life (all the pain and sufferings) and has removed the unwanted growth (an unforgiving heart and resentments). I still have "thorns," but that is the prize of my soul. I hope that you can fertilize the garden of your soul.

Finally and most important, if we want to reach heaven, we have to seek the narrow road and overcome this world. God will rejoice in our kindness toward others when we seek to give Him glory through living a life God approves of.

The way is never easy, but it is the path all good men and women must take. This was the signature line in the epic, all-time classic film The Robe.

May you all find your own way to God and into His eternal Kingdom.

"From the moment I met Julie Cox I knew she was intrinsically special person. In her heartfelt memoir, Julie scours through her past and relives her pain not for fame or fortune, but for the hope of helping others endure their sufferings with a lighter burden knowing the light shines brightly on the other side of pain. "La vida es una puta entonces we find pieces that fit together after the storm"... beautifully put, beautiful Julie"

PC Mccullough is an author, speaker and life coach. Her novel, Perfect, a story of self discovery after divorce is based on her own experiences. She has co-authored several inspirational books and co-edited the inspirational anthology, Turning Points, changing lives one event at a time.

~~~ ~~~ ~~~

"Julie Cox has written a highly compelling account of her life. Faced with many hardships at a young age, her story is one of survival through sheer pride, courage and determination. Her strength, resolve and beliefs have helped her overcome the most difficult trials of physical and mental challenges. A truly inspiring story, Julie gives us a roadmap on how we can overcome our setbacks provided we have the right attitude to succeed"

Jim Mendori is a graduate of Fordham at St.John's University in New York. He has work in the broadcasting arena as a writer, editor and political correspondent in New York, Toronto and Washington. Jim is currently a Financial Planner in NY-CT area.

~~~ ~~~ ~~~

“The first time I met Julie Cox, she asked me an interesting question. –What are you all about?” From that moment I knew I was speaking to a strong woman. She has a strong mental makeup and soul.

She has managed to overcome her challenges and become a master of her own life. In this book, she hopes many can find their own path and blueprint to success. If Julie‘s book can help one person, then she has achieved what she set out to do in the journey of helping others. That‘s Julie, that‘s what she is all about.’

Mario Ranieri is part of Nordstrom Management as well as a mentor and life coach.

~~~ ~~~ ~~~

“Two Hearts with One Mission”

I am neither a wide reader nor a good writer. But I love reading inspirational stories specially a true to life story. When I met Julie Cox, the first thing comes into my mind “is a very strong and smart woman”. The meeting of ours was not just a meeting of two different people; it was a meeting of two souls with one heart and one mission. Julie and I got a feeling of an ordinary matter in an extraordinary way of thinking that shared with love, passion and dedication and that was the connection of our hearts and the commitment of our desire in love with life and to share the inspiration not just to become famous but to share the unending inspiration about real life. Our deepest love and care for human being brought us more closely to God and the mission itself teaches us to become humble in life. When I read her story it gives me more courage to strive hard in facing struggles in life. Her book entitled “I Ordered My Future Yesterday”
~~~

was not just a collection of pains or even sufferings but it is her ways how she able to surpassed the trials in life. This book should not put only in shelves but it should be shared wherever, how far it will go.

Laila Buncajes Armamento Media Practitioner/ Freelance Writer Book Publicist/I Ordered My Future Yesterday The Julie Cox Story

~~~ ~~~ ~~~

"Flying from two opposite sides of the world, Julie Cox and I, met in the Philippines for a mission. The story of Julie Cox is a perfect epitome of "Beauty in Darkness", a documentary film which I produced. Is it possible to see the beauty in the midst of darkness? Is it possible to stay strong and keep the light of hope shining despite of the many circumstances of what seemed to be God's abandonment and condemnation by the society? Will tomorrow come after all of these? For Julie Cox, the future is in her hands. Courage, compassion and faith became her shining guide. How she overcame the challenges was beautifully written in her book. Out of darkness, she is now a successful woman who serves as an inspiration to many especially those who have lost their hope. I love you Julie. I salute you".

Aileen Collo Amparo Architect/Director Beauty in Darkness Film
~~~